How to be a Nurse
or Midwife Leade

T0176972

How to be a Nurse or Midwife Leader

Edited by

David Ashton
Director, David Ashton Development Ltd

Jamie Ripman
Director, Practive Ltd

Philippa Williams
Director, Practive Ltd

WILEY Blackwell

Library of Congress Cataloging-in-Publication Data

Names: Ashton, David, 1956– editor. | Ripman, Jamie, 1959– editor. | Williams, Philippa, editor.
Title: How to be a nurse or midwife leader / edited by David Ashton, Jamie Ripman, Philippa Williams.
Description: Chichester, West Sussex ; Hoboken, NJ : John Wiley and Sons, Ltd, 2017. | Includes bibliographical references and index.
Identifiers: LCCN 2016049509 (print) | LCCN 2016051495 (ebook) | ISBN 9781119186991 (pbk.) | ISBN 9781119187004 (pdf) | ISBN 9781119187028 (epub)
Subjects: | MESH: Nursing, Supervisory | Nurse Midwives–organization & administration | Leadership
Classification: LCC RT89 (print) | LCC RT89 (ebook) | NLM WY 105 | DDC 362.17/3068–dc23
LC record available at https://lccn.loc.gov/2016049509

A catalogue record for this book is available from the British Library.

Wiley also publishes its books in a variety of electronic formats. Some content that appears in print may not be available in electronic books.

Cover image: Meaden Creative

Set in 9.5/12pt Minion by SPi Global, Pondicherry, India

Printed in Singapore by C.O.S. Printers Pte Ltd

10 9 8 7 6 5 4 3 2 1

Contents

Authors

David Ashton, Director, David Ashton Development Ltd

Jamie Ripman, Director, Practive Ltd

Philippa Williams, Director, Practive Ltd

Caroline Alexander, Chief Nursing Officer, Bart's Health

Nicholas Bradbury, Director of Nursing & Midwifery Leadership Development, NHS Leadership Academy

James Butcher, Director, Work Without Walls

John Deffenbaugh, Director, Frontline

Catherine Eden, Director, Cumberledge Eden and Partners Ltd

Louisa Hardman, Director and Managing Consultant, Living Potential Consulting

Natilla Henry, Head of Midwifery, University College Hospitals London

Nichola Jacob, Partner, Development Potential

Nichole McIntosh, Head of Nursing, Specialty Medicine and Support Services, North Middlesex University Hospital

Michelle Mello, Deputy Director of Nursing, NHS England

Alex Pett, Director, River Leadership Consultancy Ltd

Contributors

This book would not have been possible without the generosity, wisdom and shared insights of the hundreds of nurses and midwives who attended the NHS Leadership Academy programmes in Leeds, UK, to which we refer in the book. Many of them took the time to tell us their stories of how the programme had affected their ability to lead themselves and others and so improve patient care. Through our ongoing research, we have also had contributions from other nurses and midwives who, although they didn't attend our courses in Leeds, have happily shared their stories and examples of what is possible through the deployment of the skills and strategies of leadership that we explore in the book. Unfortunately, not all of the examples have made it into these pages but we are extremely grateful to all of those who have shared their amazing stories with us:

Alison Bakewell
Alison Davidson
Alison Hughes
Angela Forster
Carmel Synan-Jones
Caroline Davies
Caroline Wilson
Christine Fawson
Clare Dikken
Clare Jones
Dawn Dawson
Dawn Marinopoulos
Emma Story
Emily Parker
Eve Scott
Fiona Wells
Gaynor Darling
Gill Findley
Gina Cook
Hayley Citrine

Helen Balsdon
Jan Glaze
Jane Ferreira
Jane Thompson
Janice Cloud
Jayne Gray
Jude Greaves-Newall
Karen Jackson
Kerry Nicholls
Kim Boormanross
Lesley Crosby
Lucy Jones
Margaret Locker
Monica Richardson
Patience Machingauta
Ruth Ostrovskis
Tania Massey
Tomasina Stacey
Tracey Carter
Val Janson

Foreword

Leadership development is an odd career to choose. You are surrounded by experts – by people with a view, a voice and some experience to share. Somewhere in the noise you need to create space for people to think, and listen and try to understand that within this field there is actually a growing body of knowledge, wisdom and expertise. The NHS Leadership Academy exists in this space – deeply proud of its work in developing leaders in health and trying hard to create space to demonstrate some wisdom and experience that contribute to what we know and can do differently in leadership. Trying to be definitive and authoritative about leadership development doesn't come easily and yet if the discipline is ever to be taken seriously then that is exactly what we have to do: to provide evidence, research and data to support our assertions about what works, what makes a difference and what can be done to learn even more.

This book is written by a group of people who are genuinely experts in their field and are sharing their wisdom through stories about a programme the Academy created for nurses and midwives working in healthcare in England. It is told with warmth and humour, is easy to read and reflects well the humanity of the authors. It draws on the experience of thousands of nurses and midwives who engaged enthusiastically in a programme of work over a two-year period which saw a coming together of some unique leadership development talent. So as you read the stories and think about the lessons shared within the pages of this book, you can rest assured that you are not just enjoying the reflections of some great practitioners but you are learning from people who really do know what they are talking about. They will help you make a difference, they will help you unlock your talent and if you are a development practitioner yourself, they will share some wonderful insights about what it really takes to create opportunities to learn creatively and make change happen.

The NHS Leadership Academy has a very simple philosophy at its heart: better leadership creates greater staff engagement which in turn creates better care. Nurses and midwives are central to this; they are the spine and sinews of an NHS providing continuously improving, high-quality, safe and compassionate care. I was deeply proud to play my part in the work of the Academy during this period and am delighted to introduce the stories of leadership at its very best in these pages. Enjoy!

Karen Lynas, Interim Managing Director, NHS Leadership Academy

Foreword

I was delighted to be asked to write a foreword for this book but deciding what to include was more difficult. There is so much I could write about from the many years I have been a nurse and a nurse leader. Nurses and midwives have so many opportunities to step into leadership roles from an early stage in their careers and you, and others, should never underestimate your impact.

A few years ago when I was the Chief Nurse in the north west of England, I came across this quote from Stephen Covey.

> *'Management is the efficiency of climbing the ladder of success. Leadership is determining whether the ladder is leaning against the right wall.'*

This had an impact on me and of course, in order to place ladders against the right walls, there are several actions and behaviours we should display, including articulating a vision or direction, creating opportunities, inspiring, encouraging and enabling others, and now, more than ever before, creating, nurturing and sustaining relationships.

Writing this in 2016, we are facing many complex challenges with very significant pressures on the health and care sector. This makes the quote used in the introduction to this book so important.

> *'Adaptive leadership is the practice of mobilizing people to tackle tough challenges and thrive.'*

As we have set out in our Nursing, Midwifery and Care Staff Framework *Leading Change, Adding Value* (May 2016), every nurse and midwife is a leader and has a key role in leading the response to the challenges of today while also determining the future. My vision is for our professions to take the lead, collaborating with others to determine the best way to deliver health and care that can adapt and respond to the needs of our population.

To do that, we should first discover ourselves. This is not about being self-indulgent or navel gazing but critical to understanding our impact on others, how we respond under pressure and how we treat our colleagues. If we are authentic, we are more credible.

Telling stories, providing examples and describing personal experiences can be inspirational and will engage with colleagues and those we want to influence. This book has many real examples and will no doubt have more of a lasting impact on you than theory and fine words.

As you read this book, think about your 'lollipop moments', when someone you worked with, or for, said or did something that had a significant impact on how you do your job or how you behave. Over the years, I have been lucky enough to have a few of those moments – from the ward sister who ran the first ward I worked on as a student, the nursing officer who gave me permission to introduce something new on the ward when I was a staff nurse, the clinical nurse specialist who supported my husband when he had leukemia and my boss when I worked at the Department of Health. In their different ways, they and others helped shape my decisions and showed me the importance of leading others with skill.

Traditional professional and organisational boundaries are also inappropriate in the current and future context. Our patients and the people we support and care for need us to communicate and collaborate across our complex systems in order to deliver the changes we need. In your career, take opportunities to work in different settings.

This book provides you with theory but also, importantly, practical advice on how to be a nurse or midwifery leader. Take opportunities, look for opportunities and inspire others to do the same. Together we can respond to the challenges of today but crucially lead the development and design of the future health and care system.

Jane Cummings, Chief Nursing Officer for England

Introduction

'There are almost as many different definitions of leadership as there are persons who have attempted to define the concept.' (Bass, 1981)

At the time of writing, if you google the word 'leadership', you get 629 000 000 responses. Similarly, if you search for books on leadership, you will find 369 000 000 suggestions. Over the past 50 or so years, there has been an explosion of research, discussion, debate and analysis of what constitutes leadership.

If you've picked up this book, we assume you've got an interest at least! And that, depending on where you are in your career as a nurse or midwife, you also might be thinking to yourself, 'Am I a leader?' or 'In what way am I a leader?'.

So we thought it would be helpful to start by outlining what we mean by leadership, why we think it's important and how we hope this book can help you. We could spend a long time word-smithing another addition to the many definitions of leadership. However, we find Ronald Heifetz's description of what he calls 'adaptive leadership' a helpful one.

'Adaptive leadership is the practice of mobilizing people to tackle tough challenges and thrive.' (Heifetz et al., 2009)

The word 'adaptive' here acknowledges the importance of how context determines the leadership challenges that we face. Simply put, the world keeps changing and we need to be able to respond to those changes. Very importantly, this definition is not about leadership role or position but about the activity, or practice, and the impact – notice the word 'thrive' here. So implicit in this, we believe, is the notion that we can lead from wherever we are in any organisation or system, whatever our responsibilities or job title. Benjamin Zander and Rosamund Stone Zander, in their book *The Art of Possibility* (2000), define this as 'leading from any chair'. Throughout this book, we offer examples of when nurses and midwives have demonstrated leadership at all levels and in many different contexts. This includes the newly qualified nurse who challenges a senior consultant on his behaviour to a patient, the staff nurse who introduced a change to mental health practice, the group of nurses who sought to change practice around care given to orthopaedic patients and many more besides.

If we can agree that this is a good enough definition of the task of leadership, our aim in this book is to explore what it takes to lead well – the 'how' of the title. Before we do that, let's get back to the notion that the context in which we live, work and lead provides the challenges we face – as human beings and as leaders. This connects to the 'why' of leadership; Victor Frankl (2004) famously said 'Those who have a "why" to live can bear with almost any "how"'. As we'll discuss later in the book, for example in Chapters 1 and 3, we believe a fundamental part of the 'how' of leadership is being in touch with the 'why': why are you doing this, for what purpose, in whose interests are you acting?

So why do *we* think that leadership for nurses and midwives is so important? As we write this book, we are living in difficult times. At a global level, there are humanitarian disasters on an unimaginable scale as thousands of people seek refuge from their own war-torn or poverty-stricken countries. This runs alongside global financial crises; whether we have just come out of or are about to go back into a recession is a moot point, and not within the scope of this book. But we can certainly say that many people are suffering from times of austerity and that there is a huge challenge for healthcare as the NHS and other providers struggle with less money, not enough qualified people and increasing demand. And yet at the centre of the NHS lies a great purpose, articulated in the NHS Constitution.

> 'The NHS belongs to the people. It is there to improve our health and well-being, supporting us to keep mentally and physically well, to get better when we are ill and, when we cannot fully recover, to stay as well as we can until the end of our lives … The NHS is founded on a common set of principles and values that bind together the communities and people it serves, patients and public and the staff who work for it. It touches our lives at times of basic human need when care and compassion are what matter most.' (Department of Health, 2015)

We appreciate that some of you reading this may not be working directly for the NHS. But we should nail our colours to the mast here and say that we hope this aspiration also reflects the aspirations of *all* healthcare professionals whether they work for the NHS, a commercial provider or a social enterprise, not least because the future may look very different indeed in terms of the organisation of healthcare provision. We acknowledge this is not an easy 'ask' and we think that all nurses and midwives (as indeed all healthcare professionals) have a personal responsibility and accountability to be the best leader they can be in the service of delivering outstanding patient care.

This book is sponsored by the NHS Leadership Academy and came about after a series of leadership development programmes run by the Academy for nurses and midwives from 2012 to 2016. Through these programmes, and other multiprofessional leadership programmes, at the time of writing, the Academy has worked with over 10 000 nurses and midwives from frontline staff to senior nurses. At the centre of the nursing and midwifery leadership programmes was the principle that if 'care and compassion are what matter most', then nurses and midwives are at the very heart of that, and their leadership is what will continue to help bring about this eloquently expressed ambition in the very challenging times in which we find ourselves.

So we in turn are ambitious for this book; we believe great leadership is what will help the NHS, and the provision of healthcare in all its forms, adapt, survive and remain resilient for future generations.

Practical

Given all of the above, this book is intended to be practical; whilst underpinned by academic theory, the emphasis is on application – the 'how to' of the title. In keeping with this, the chapters all contain exercises and/or reflective or provocative questions to get you thinking about the application of the theory to your leadership. So we encourage you to take time out, pause and reflect, do the exercises and explore the questions. However much we know, it is how we use and embody that knowledge, live it and breathe it that determines the impact of our leadership. Trying out the exercises will better equip you to be able to translate leadership theory into leadership practice.

The book is aimed at all nurses and midwives who wish to develop and improve their practice as leaders. In that practical spirit, our hope is that it can be a companion which you can refer to at different points in your careers, from third-year students about to embark on your first newly qualified roles, to stepping into a team leader role, to leading a ward, to leading a service.

Grounded in reality

Through the work we have done with the Leadership Academy, we have been able to capture many real-life examples of leadership in practice from nurses and midwives across the system. This means that this book is absolutely grounded in the detailed reality of lived experience. It takes note of the many different situations in which you work. We've already talked about how leadership challenges are driven by the context; by this we mean both the ever xvi **Introduction**

changing political, social and environmental context and the individual contexts in which you find yourselves. We understand that, for example, the world of a ward sister in a large acute London trust is very different from that of a community midwife in a rural area, and different again from a role in a care home or mental health trust. These contexts provide different leadership challenges, which in turn may require different leadership responses.

The human, personal and relational

The book focuses on the human, personal and relational aspects of leadership, rather than the clinical and technical aspects of nursing and midwifery, exploring the question, 'what do I need to know and how do I need to be as a human being to be an effective and successful leader who can improve and deliver patient-focused care?'.

Three core principles have helped us to shape the content. Put simply, in order to be the best leaders we can be, we need to lead ourselves well, lead others with skill and lead collectively and collaboratively outside traditional boundaries. These three elements overlap; in graphic terms you might represent them as a Venn diagram.

However, we start where we think leadership has to begin – with an inquiry into ourselves – how have I become the person and leader I am and what kind of leader do I aspire to be? In Part 1, 'Leading myself well', we explore how to develop self-awareness, how to understand the impact we have on others ('What's it like to be on the receiving end of me?') and how to look after ourselves in order to be able to look after others.

Part 2 then looks to how we work with others – building relationships of trust, leading one conversation at a time, communicating to different audiences, influencing with integrity, motivating and getting the best out of others.

Part 3 broadens the scope to explore a leader's responsibility to see beyond their organisational and professional silos, to build collective and collaborative leadership across the system, working with complexity, helping to build a compassionate, diverse and inclusive culture, navigating the politics and looking to co-create the future of healthcare.

Cross-cutting themes

Of course, leadership, like life, can't always be fitted into neat categories, so you will definitely see some recurring themes that cut across all the sections. These include the fundamental need for self-awareness; 'authenticity' – what that means and how you can 'be yourself well in all situations'; the notion that leadership happens 'one conversation at a time'; the need, in all those conversations, to be skilful both at enquiring into others' views ('seek first to understand') and advocating your own; the importance of diversity and inclusion.

The importance of diversity and inclusion

Our intention is that, in keeping with the practical nature of this book, you will find the style engaging and conversational. You will also notice that the chapters have their own unique 'voices'. We've already established that leadership is a bit of a contested field and that there are as many different views and opinions about good leadership as there are human beings. Diversity of thinking, background and experience is fundamental to any successful human enterprise and we believe that a key part of leadership is to go outside your own comfort zone, seek different views and include those who are different from you. For those who work in public bodies like the NHS, this is of course a statutory responsibility; the NHS Constitution has this as its first principle.

> 'The NHS provides a comprehensive service, available to all irrespective of gender, race, disability, age, sexual orientation, religion, belief, gender reassignment, pregnancy and maternity or marital or civil partnership status. The service is designed to diagnose, treat and improve both physical and mental health. It has a duty to each and every individual that it serves and must respect human rights.' (Department of Health, 2015)

For us, this goes beyond a statutory responsibility; it is about who we are as human beings.

> 'If we can work openly and honestly with our differences. If we can embrace them and have the difficult conversations that all good relationships have, then we can create possibilities that we cannot yet conceive of. We can create the possibility of us evolving organisations that are truly "fit to house the human spirit".' (Dr Eden Charles, unpublished, 2014)

In keeping with the spirit of diversity, we have sought different contributors for this book, who bring differing perspectives and who speak with their own voices and write in their own style. As you read, notice your response to the different styles: which voices do you warm to, which styles do you prefer, which do you find less easy to relate to (if any)? Then, importantly, ask yourself what that preference tells you about you! And how might those preferences affect the way you communicate with and lead others who are different from you?

Our hope and our aim are that this book can inspire, motivate and help resource nurse and midwife leaders in service of delivering and improving the very best patient care, in collaboration with the thousands of dedicated and talented staff of the NHS.

References

Bass, B.M. (1981) *Sodgill's Handbook of Leadership: a survey of theory and research.* New York: Free Press.

Department of Health (2015) *The NHS Constitution for England.* London: Department of Health.

Heifetz, R.A., Grashow, A. and Linsky, M. (2009) *The Practice of Adaptive Leadership: tools and tactics for changing your organization and the world.* Boston, MA: Harvard Business School Press.

Frankl, V.E. (2004) *Man's Search for Meaning.* London: Rider.

Zander, B. and Zander, R.S. (2000) *The Art of Possibility: transforming professional and personal life.* Boston, MA: Harvard Business School Press.

Part 1

Leading myself well

Chapter 1 **To begin at the beginning ...**

David Ashton

Identity and self at work

The subject of identity at work is complex and can be viewed from a whole range of different perspectives. It is important that we have an understanding of this so that we can appreciate different views of what it means and feels like to be at work and as nurses and midwives why we do what we do.

This chapter will take you through some of the theoretical aspects of identity, specifically identity in the context of work and also in the context of being part of a profession. The professions of nursing and midwifery can represent, through the work they do, all that is best about the NHS and society more broadly. Society places trust and an expectation on the people in these roles that they will be technically capable and proficient and equally able to deliver that technical capability in a kind and compassionate way. The profession holds something for the collective societal psyche so when tragedies occur, such as the appalling failings in care at Mid-Staffordshire NHS Trust, they undermine the trust that has been hard won and afforded by society and the best efforts of those committed to excellence in care delivery. 'Kindness is not a side issue, it is what we are about and it is what leadership is about' (Ballatt and Campling, 2011). Or as one nurse put it:

> *'The technical work of nursing is one thing, of course it can be emotionally difficult and demanding. Leading a team to maintain compassion in care is another matter… it's what I've signed up to do, it's what I will do… otherwise why bother? You've got to be technically up to the job and you've got to be emotionally literate, attuned.'* (Ward Sister, acute trust)

In this chapter we will address the notion of how we, and others, might see ourselves as nurses and midwives and specifically as leaders in those professions.

How to be a Nurse or Midwife Leader, First Edition.
Edited by David Ashton, Jamie Ripman and Philippa Williams.
© 2017 John Wiley & Sons, Ltd. Published 2017 by John Wiley & Sons, Ltd.

We will also explore something of what it means to be a professional. The following vignette refers to the aunt of the chapter author and illustrates the deep attachment of one person to her professional identity – the story of one individual that can be applied to many people.

Edie and the story of is/was.

Edie, my aunt, is/was a nurse. She had been a ward sister in what was termed a psychiatric hospital, in fact her mother had also been a sister at the same hospital and her father had been a charge nurse there. As a nurse I broke the mould a little, but only a little, I was a registered general nurse, my wife was a nurse and midwife and one of our daughters was a dental nurse… as you see, it runs in the family. A family tradition that isn't that uncommon in nursing or in fact other professions and occupations.

*At the time of writing this, Edie was in a state of is/was being a nurse. Again, at the time of writing, she was 86 years old and had dementia. As many of you will know, this cruel disease, which gradually corrupts then wipes your memory, was little by little taking her away from herself and the people around her, at first disconnecting her personal and social constructs, then moving around and finally removing the pieces of her personal and social jigsaw. Yet her identity and recollections of her time working as a nurse are a common touching place in our conversations, somewhere where her memories are clear and still have meaning. The is/was comes into play because there are times when she knows she **was** a ward sister, she recounts incidents both good and bad accurately, the level of detail and recall is accurate and focused. When ex-colleagues come to visit, she knows who they are and what they did. There are also times when she still **is** the ward sister, she talks as if she is on duty, at times referring to the other care home residents as her patients, admonishing the staff if she thinks they are late with meals and then praising them for something she has approved of. By and large people go with the **was** and **is** quite readily – it regulates everyone. I think there is something helpful about sharing common ground and looking through a window at a shared memory of what was and who she was.*

We, the family, fill her room with artefacts of her past, including a picture of Edie and her mother, my grandmother, resplendent in starched hats and cuffs, big silver buckles gleaming on blue belts – and to be frank looking pretty forbidding! She takes pride in this and refers to it often – it is a powerful connection to her mother and their shared identity. The very way they stand in the photograph speaks of their professional position and their pride in it. For my part, when Edie first arrived in the care home, I too was keen to make sure the staff knew she had been a nurse and had also cared for people with dementia.

The relevance of this story in the context of this book is that Edie's identity as a nurse still matters to her, it matters to the author and it matters as information to the staff and how they relate to Edie as someone in their care. Until recently, when her condition deteriorated, it mattered to some of the other residents as she tried to organise them in her role as 'ward sister'! Her state of is/was is a story of her identity and whilst there are other aspects to her personal construct, her identity as a nurse is hugely significant – it forms part of her psyche, the essence of who she is. There is often something very important to people, especially people whose role sits somewhere on a spectrum of a calling or vocation at one end and a transactional paid-for or waged task at the other. And, like Edie, it can be one of the most significant aspects of their personal construct. This nurse's description of going back to work after a career break captures the excitement of returning to her calling beautifully.

'"Nursing is the art of caring" – a tutor told me that when I first started my training and I've always treasured it. I'd had a break from nursing while my children were small, and was so excited to return to the bedside. I had missed the action, the passion and that great feeling of making a difference. The night before I could barely sleep – I was back to where I wanted to be. I couldn't wait to put my medal back on.' (Unit Co-ordinator of a frail care unit, BUPA)

First impressions and identity

It's pretty common in a social setting for people to introduce themselves by their name, fairly obvious really, not to mention immensely helpful. However, the introduction is frequently followed by a question, particularly when meeting someone for the first time, and that question usually goes something like 'and so, what do you do?'. At one level this is a pleasantry, a show of interest to find out more about the person you have just met. There is also a deeper reason, a question behind the question if you like, something of which the questioner may not even be consciously aware. Why we do this is pretty complex but the reason can be that we need to place the other person somewhere in the social structure or, more specifically, somewhere in the social structure in relation to ourselves – it's a social anthropologist's field day!

Make a note of this 'and so what do you do?' the next time you're in a social setting – try and gauge the other person's response and reactions, and just as importantly, note your own! Notice what you feel as well as what you think. If, like me, you're a people watcher, see how other people interact.

The reality is that our decisions about who the other person is generally start before any words are spoken at all. Depending on our senses, we might make an assessment of the other person's gender, ethnicity, sexuality, age, language or accent, their smell, their attractiveness, their clothing, mannerisms, etc.; a whole range of data is taken in and processed. Some of us more than others will then start to formulate judgements, make assumptions, position the individual by social grouping, putting them into one or more social categories. Our known, and also our unconscious, biases will kick in, arousing different types of emotion both positive and negative and whether the other person is more or less like us; are they part of our 'in-group' or do they belong to some other 'out-group'? Another reason the 'and so, what do you do?' question is asked is that the questioner is really more interested in telling you about themselves, their achievements, their status. They may, in fact, not be that interested in what *you* do; they aren't on receive; they are much more invested in telling you what *they* do. They are on transmit and seeking to impose their social standing, their level and sources of power, their ego. In effect, it's about superiority and privilege.

We know also that privilege, bias and discrimination can be barriers in colleague-to-colleague relationships that can have direct and negative effects on patient care. This has been increasingly evidenced by the work of Dawson (2009, 2014), Kline (2014) and West *et al.* (2011). The relevance here is that we need to understand our personal construct, to help us understand the perspective of others and how we can interact positively; we all have prejudices and biases. As mentioned previously, this applies to difference in relation to minority groups in their broadest sense and particularly to those who are visibly different from the majority. Black and minority ethnic (BME) colleagues and BME people receiving care can face more challenging barriers to their personal identity than those of the majority group. The adoption across the NHS of the Workforce Race Equality Standard (WRES) is testament to the amount that needs to be done to improve matters in relation to diversity and inclusion in the NHS. As this book is being written, the WRES is in its very early days and it will be crucially important for improved patient care that its adoption is supported by deeper organisational development work across the NHS if the care system is to become a place that is truly inclusive for staff and, importantly, for the people receiving care.

If you haven't looked at it already, get a copy of Roger Kline's paper 'The "snowy white peaks" of the NHS'. It's well worth considering how this impacts you, or not. Discuss it with colleagues and think about your reaction to this as you continue your leadership journey.

Our attempts to work out our social fit also depend on context – it's one thing at a party, it would be different in the street and it is different again in a work setting and particularly so when that work setting involves the mental and physical health of others – what Strauss *et al.* (1982) referred to as 'sentimental work':

> '*Sentimental work is an ingredient in any kind of work where the object being worked on is alive, sentient, reacting an ingredient either because deemed necessary to get the work done effectively or because of humanistic considerations. Sentimental work has its source in the elementary fact that work done with or on human beings may have to take into account their responses to that instrumental work (as with medical work); indeed their responses may be a central feature of that work.*' (Strauss *et al.*, 1982, p. 254)

The point here is that definitions of what constitutes our work identity and a simple 'and so, what do you do?' are not simple at all. We need to understand these constructs as we develop as leaders – we may have spent many years training and honing our technical skills to be highly competent practitioners, a journey which will continue through our working lives. For some of us our professional identity will be a large part of our personal construct (Kelly, 1953) – it may in part define who we are in the world, it holds something of the essence of who we are and purport to be. At other times it is more background as other identities, or aspects of our identity, come to the fore.

There is a huge amount of literature and many schools of thought that explore the notion of self and identity in society; you may well have covered much of this during training and since qualification, particularly in relation to health and ill health. There is equally a large body of literature that covers the subject of self and identity in relation to work, both paid and unpaid. Much of this is beyond the remit of this book but it might be helpful to touch on a couple of definitions about self and identity in relation to work roles.

The author Ashforth (2001) suggests that we define our work roles and identity using two different perspectives, and although the terms and descriptions themselves seem at first sight to be complex, they provide a helpful lens through which to make sense of the differing approaches to identity at work.

- *Structural functionalism* – a theoretical approach stemming from the work of Emile Durkheim which suggests that we enact our role based on a whole range of socially constructed norms. This is particularly true for people in 'professional' roles where there is a historical identified norm – teachers, nurses, the police. As relationships with the recipients of 'care' change, along with the standing of professionals and the professions in society, this equilibrium of relationship is being challenged, and often rightly so.

- *Symbolic interactionism* – the basis of this is that roles are an emergent and negotiated understanding between individuals. This is based on Blumer (1969) and Mead's (1934) work and not dissimilar to the internal dialogue described from a psychological perspective by Kelly (1953) in personal construct theory. This approach acknowledges much more the subjective, interactive and fluid nature of co-created social and psychological relationships, the self being shaped by social interaction (Hogg and Vaughan, 2006, p. 116).

You might ask why these definitions matter. I would suggest that the first construct, structural functionalism, speaks to the historical past of how our profession is seen. As mentioned previously, this might be for better or worse. The second construct, symbolic interactionism, provides both opportunity and threat. We, the system, society, have an opportunity to generate a new identity – a co-created state. Where professionals and the people we are employed to work with, our patients and clients, negotiate our identities. Moving from a paternalistic model of care to one where openness and responsibility are shared.

Professional power and responsibility

It is also helpful to consider for a moment what we mean by a profession. Again, there are many definitions but here are a couple to play around with. First, Fish and Coles (1998) restated Friedson's definition of a profession as:

- *An occupation exercising 'good' in the service of another*
- *Specialised work in that it cannot entirely be understood by the layman*
- *Not measured by financial reward alone*
- *Ethically and morally based*
- *Having an esoteric and complex knowledge base*
- *Exercising discretion*
- *Dependent upon professional judgement.*

Or this by Miller *et al.* (2002, p. 26) who suggest that a profession has:

- *A high degree of self-regulation*
- *Activities founded on an abstract body of knowledge*
- *Entry to the profession controlled by qualification and certification*
- *A private language that serves both to unify the group and mystify others*
- *Claims of exclusive competence to carry out certain types of work*
- *A set of values, often made explicit in a code of ethics.*

It's worth noting that in these definitions there are some positive qualities as well as some that are much less flattering, particularly in relation to language and how it can be used to mystify others. A number of authors have written about differences in power and authority both within and between professions. In his writings about the sociological development of the medical profession, Friedson (1970, p. 72) noted that 'the work of one professional group overlaps, even competes with that of other occupations', and he goes on to comment that:

> '*A profession attains and maintains its position by virtue of the protection and patronage of some elite segment of society which is persuaded that there is some special value in its work. Its position is thus secured by the political and economic influence of the elite which sponsors it – an influence that drives competing occupations out of the same area of work, that discourages others by virtue of the competitive advantages conferred by the chosen occupation, and that requires still others to be subordinated to the profession.*' (Friedson, 1972, p. 72)

Lingard *et al.* (2003, p. 614) discuss this as a world-view held by one clinical group about another where clinical colleagues are described as 'others' and 'unreliable enemies' in the competition for authority and resources. Ferlie and Geraghty (2007) note this as a phenomenon across the UK public sector more generally.

> '*The relationship between professional groups is as important as that between professionals and managers. The public sector contains an extensive range of professional groupings. Dominant professionals typically seek to marginalise the jurisdictions of subordinate professions.*' (Ferlie and Geraghty, 2007, p. 426)

If you want to know more about this in relationship to 'the professions' in general, look up Eliot Friedson, who did much research and wrote extensively about the sociology of the professions, or Guggenbuhl-Craig (2015) who covers power in therapeutic relationships.

As an exercise, talk to colleagues and, if you can, people who don't work in nursing or midwifery, and see what terms they would use to describe their profession – do they in fact actually view it as one?

There are challenges as you develop as a leader. First, how do you hold onto your credibility as a clinician, something probably very dear to your heart, as your leadership responsibilities increase? Second, does your very identity as a nurse or midwife act as a boundary to your acceptance by other groups, including other professionals, and is it something that might in fact be a barrier to developments and improvements in patient care? These two quotes suggest these are points worthy of consideration.

> '... a *"supra-non-profession"*: that is, an occupation which has emerged from the ranks of the professionals, to run the profession from a managerial rather than a professional perspective. The irony, as we shall see, is that enhanced status is dependent on managerial rather than professional expertise.' (Healy and Kraithman, 1996, p. 188)

> 'The problem is one of managing elites. Each profession tends to regard itself as an elite.Members look to their profession and to their peers to determine codes of behaviour and acceptable performance standards. They often disdain the values and evaluations of those outside their discipline ... Most professionals are reluctant to subordinate themselves to others, or to support organisational goals not completely congruent with their special viewpoint.' (Quinn et al., 1996, p. 11)

If these points are valid, and experience suggests that this can be the case, we have a responsibility to be mindful of this for our own practice as leaders and also the practice of others. Equally, rather than being suspicious of the motives of other groups, we need to maintain a curiosity and openness that allow the possibility of different approaches that encourage creativity and innovation – to paraphrase a well-known saying, 'no profession is an island'.

As a nurse or midwife, you are subject to a range of emotions – it's the nature and substance of the job, it's ever present in what we do. As you evolve as a leader, this will become more complex. As mentioned earlier, you will continue to evolve as a clinician, so too will you evolve as a leader. Diagrammatically, a typical career journey may go something like Figure 1.1.

One ward sister noted that:

> 'I sometimes get more anxious, nervous, when dealing with managerial issues. They can be more costly – you know I get physiological symptoms. One minute you have to pull someone up about a performance issue and the next minute you're asking them a favour, to work an extra shift or something. I have to do a lot of steeling inside.' (Ward Sister, acute trust)

The notion of leadership, how best to lead and the tools and techniques of leadership will be constant themes throughout this book. It is also important to consider as an individual who you are as a nurse or midwife, your position not only within the profession but also society more broadly. I mentioned earlier that the meaning we make of work can sit somewhere on a continuum

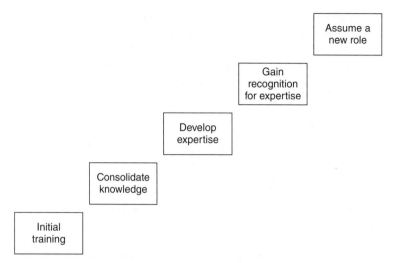

Figure 1.1 Role transition ladder.

between a calling or vocation and a paid-for or waged task. The reality is that at times it may feel like one thing and at others it will take on a different meaning in our lives as personal priorities change. We will look at this in two stages: first, we will explore what it means to be a professional and second, we will delve into personal identity and how the changes in your role might affect your identity.

The 'professions' have arguably come under an increasing level of scrutiny over recent years. No longer is it sufficient to say that the nurse, the doctor, the teacher, the solicitor knows best. That said, even in his 1906 play *The Doctor's Dilemma*, George Bernard Shaw castigated the professions as 'a conspiracy at the expense of the laity',

This at times rather messy interprofessional dynamic can be further compounded by what Lord Rose, in his review of leadership in the NHS, refers to as the 'balkanization of trusts and silo working'. In his words:

> '*There are currently 211 CCGs, 158 Acute Trusts, 10 Ambulance Trusts, 51 Mental Health Trusts and 31 Health and Care Trusts as part of the NHS federation as well as a myriad of other providers of care. The landscape of this federation has become fragmented in terms of both the numbers and activities of Trusts; within many Trusts silo working is endemic. This means that any activity within a Trust is horizontally separated from the same activity in other Trusts and vertically separated from other activities in its home Trust.*

> *The same is true for CCGs, where there is a need for greater local and regional collaboration. Yet collaboration is more difficult in an environment that has been designed to create competition. Better communication between Trusts and CCGs would help reduce fragmentation of the landscape. There are too many "city-states" and not enough cooperation between them.'* (Department of Health, 2015, pp. 42–43)

While it might seem that these system-level or interprofessional tangles belong elsewhere, their effect can be systemic and, more importantly, they can have an impact on day-to-day patient care. As someone in a leadership role or about to take on leadership responsibilities, it is important that you develop an understanding of the organisational and professional geographies around you. That way, you can better understand the context in which you work and also how to inform it in a positive way. As your career as a leader progresses, so too do the scope and breadth of your responsibility and accountability; this in turn can be matched by your levels of influence and authority. These latter two factors – influence and authority – can be utilised for good or ill to exert power and control. This is an emotive area and many will already recognise, and have experienced, the well-known phrase 'power corrupts; absolute power corrupts absolutely'.

As someone nearing the end of their training, you should consider the increasing responsibilities you hold, and also how you will utilise the corresponding influence and authority this carries with it.

Those who have been qualified for some time will be aware of the added tensions this can bring – some of these challenges and opportunities will be addressed later in this book.

It's worth considering for a moment how to acknowledge and access the different sources of power at your disposal; those that you have experienced and those that you have knowingly, or indeed unknowingly, exercised. There are many variations on the model used here to suggest sources of power but this list, taken from Pedler *et al.* (2003), is a helpful place to start. It is also worth considering these in relation to the leadership styles referred to in Chapter 4 to see if there is any crossover.

There are three types of position power.

- *Role power* – derives from your role and status and the perception that you have the right to exercise influence because of this. This kind of power is linked to the hierarchical structure of an organisation and defines the scope of your authority.

- *Coercive power* – is based on the use of fear. It depends upon other people thinking that you can punish them if they do not comply. Examples of this might include strong measures such as formal reprimands, the withdrawal of promotion or privileges, the allocation of unpleasant duties and even dismissal. But there are many highly effective and subtler forms of coercion such as disapproval, withdrawal of friendship, exclusion from key meetings.
- *Reward power* – the twin of coercion, the carrot to go with the stick. Reward power is based on the perception that you have the ability and resources to reward the compliant. There are many ways to reward people including praise, recognition, increased responsibilities and the granting of individual privileges. Pay or promotion or the allocation of 'desirable' work are other possibilities.

There are also three types of personal power.

- *Expert power* – based on your competence or special knowledge in a given area. Expert power is based on credibility, and the value attached to the particular field in which you can show competence.
- *Referent power* – based on the influence that comes from your personal attractiveness to others. It is the power which arises from your personal characteristics and charisma, your reputation, and the respect of others or esteem in which you are held.
- *Connection power* – derives from networks and relationships. This kind of power can be used to build political knowledge, gather information, gain personal support and feedback or build trust and alliances. This source of power is becoming ever more relevant in a networked workplace and through the increasing use of social media.

This isn't an exhaustive list and you could certainly alter the definitions somewhat. However, it illustrates the fact that power, influence and control can be used negatively as well as positively. It is within your gift as you develop as a leader to determine how you use them.

> As an exercise, either with peers or with a supervisor, have a conversation about occasions when you have experienced the use/misuse of power. Think also about times when you might have avoided the use of your own power when it might have been more appropriate to exercise it.
>
> As mentioned power can be a term that evokes a negative reaction - what other terms might you use?

Before finishing this section, I want to focus in particular on the use or, possibly from my observations, denial of two aspects of power mentioned above – the 'twins' of power *coercion* and *reward*.

Twins appear frequently in many cultures – Apollo and Artemis, Hypnos and Thanatos, Freya and Freyr. They are sometimes portrayed as the alter ego of each other, an aspect of the self that we might prefer to keep out of view, hidden or in the shadow, even out of our own view. So too in leadership and the life of work teams and organisations in general. Most of us will have come across the work of Carl Jung; Hede (2007) picks up on his writings and works with the notion of the shadow in exploring the negative side of emotions in work groups – this shadow or twin he calls the shadow self. The overt self is those characteristics and qualities which we are aware of and that we use to self-define ourselves and reveal to others. On the other hand, our shadow self is the part of our psyche that we do not readily recognise in ourselves and that we may project onto others.

- Our overt self – in our awareness
  - defines us to ourselves
  - reveals us to others
  - manages our interactions
- Our shadow self – out of awareness
  - opposite of overt self
  - qualities of our self that we do not accept.
  - projected on to others

The link to coercion and reward is of particular relevance to privilege and specifically how some people in society are more privileged than others – we need to seriously consider this as clinicians in relation to the patients we work with and particularly so as leaders. There is a great deal of evidence that describes how minority groups are excluded from certain privileges; we tend to privilege those who are like us. This may not be a conscious act but it exists – it often resides in our shadow self and leads to the creation of excluded individuals and groups and those who are included. Our society is a male-gendered hegemony – that is, men tend to hold positional power, role power in our earlier model, and the NHS is no exception to this (Beardwell and Holden, 1997).

As you evolve as a leader, part of your role will be to hold a line in relation to acceptable and unacceptable behaviours – someone once said that 'we judge ourselves by our intentions and we judge others by their actions or behaviours'. This clearly applies to activities that sit within the clinical realm of your practice; however, as importantly, your responsibility will increasingly become ever more salient in the managerially focused aspect of your leadership role. The gravitas and personal authority you portray will become more visible and an increasing part of who you are at work. If you work and live in a community setting, and are known by neighbours and your broader community, the 'segmentation' of work identity and non-work identity becomes ever more blurred; this is where the definitions of 'structural functionalism' and 'symbolic interactionism' come into their own. Your 'professional self' and your 'personal' or 'private self' become ever more merged. This can be applied to anyone whose role is publicly visible in their community such as teachers, social workers and the police – community workers in the broadest sense of the term.

Roles and role transition

Does our role or job define who we are, or do we define our role or job? Maybe you view it as a vocation? One reality is that as our careers progress, particularly as clinicians and people who are paid to care, the expectations that others have of us will change. The expectations placed on you as someone in training will be very different from those placed on you as a qualified person. The moment you put on a different style of uniform and your name badge has a different title, you will be different – or will you? You're still pretty much the same you as you were the day before. What has changed, though, – other people's perception, be they patients or colleagues, and very probably our own perception.

In life, we have a whole range of roles beyond those that are work related. Some are defined by our position in our family: mother, son, sister, aunt, stepfather, etc. Others by our connection to social groups, for example political party member, netball team member, social class, ethnic group, and also our position within that social grouping, such as party leader, secretary, head chorister, alto, soprano, team captain, wing defence, wing attack, etc. So too at work we have formal job titles that denote our position and give us some level of formal authority or power. This collection of identities or self-images is referred to as our 'role set' (Katz and Khan, 1978). However, in a work setting we also occupy a host of other informal roles or duties; some of us may be seen as more nurturing of others, some as holding the organisation's or team's knowledge and history, some as holding the real source of power in the team. It's a key leadership skill to identify and work with the people whose names may not appear on an organisation's organogram, which links back to the earlier point about sources of personal and positional power.

> An organogram is the pictorial representation of an organisation's structure, often set out in a hierarchical way. Take a look at your organisation or team structure and who holds what sort of power – you could compare this with who in reality impacts on your sphere of work and who doesn't appear on the chart. Lastly, consider where you might feature and how you use your sources of power.

Leadership, power and emotional work

> '*Emotion! Most of my work is dealing with staff problems, involved in dealing with people's emotion and the problems people have at work and at home. You have to do emotion work – it doesn't just apply to patients. But being emotional isn't all negative, you have to be in touch with the real world, sometimes it hurts but you shouldn't split it off.*' (Senior Sister, accident and emergency)

So to end this chapter, I will touch on leading in an emotional workspace. As our roles change and we become clinically more proficient, the potential for our standing as a leader increases; remember the links to sources of power. Leaders can be good and they can also be bad – the NHS has some excellent leaders at many levels and there are some examples of poor leadership too. However, a particular and unique responsibility is placed on those people who lead in a world where the very nature of the work is with sentient beings – there is an emotional aspect to what we do. This applies in many walks of life where the employee is paid to care; you can read more broadly about this in the seminal work of Arlie Hochschild, called *The Managed Heart*. In short, Hochschild made observations of people who were paid to 'care' and she coined the term 'emotional work', something she defined as follows.

> '*Emotional work is the effort we put into ensuring that our private feelings are suppressed or represented to be in tune with socially accepted norms – such as looking happy and enthusiastic at a friend's party, when we actually feel tired and bored. Emotional labour is the commercial exploitation of this principle; when an employee is in effect paid to smile, laugh, be polite, or be caring.*' (Hochschild, 1983, p. 7)

To paraphrase the NHS Constitution, 'when that work touches lives at times of basic human need, when care and compassion are what matter most', that work assumes a different level of gravitas. In a wonderful book by John Ballatt and Penelope Campling, they reframe the notion of work as the application of 'intelligent kindness', saying that:

> '*It is a binding, creative and problem-solving force that inspires and focusses the imagination and goodwill. It inspires and directs the attention and efforts of people and organisations towards building relationships with patients, recognising their needs and treating them well. Kindness is not a "nice" side issue in the project of competitive progress. It is the "glue" of cooperation required for such progress to be the most benefit to most people.*' (Ballatt and Campling, 2011, p. 16)

Finally, to go back to Edie for a moment, she wrote a piece in the final in-house magazine to be published on the closure of a psychiatric hospital she had worked at. Some of her thoughts and opinions may be of a different time and others may have a different view from her, but I believe some of her opinions have relevance for today. She believed in tolerance of others, she believed powerfully that those with a duty of care should practise professionally and knowledgeably. Above all, she felt that care wasn't something that existed solely in the domain of the 'professional' – it was a societal responsibility. She wrote this when the hospital closed in 1989:

'I was one of our family's second generation at Broadgate [Hospital, nr Beverley in East Yorkshire]. My parents worked there as well as my brother and uncle.

The closure of Broadgate is very sad, but we are now entering an exciting time for psychiatry. It remains to be seen whether society will give the care that has been promised. I realise nothing can remain at a standstill, but a nice hospital has gone. It was one of the better ones – in my view unique.

I had 20 years [working] in acute psychiatry from 1950 to 1970 and feel that this was the period of biggest change. These were the years when they let us unlock the doors. I witnessed the introduction of psychiatric drugs which had a profound effect on the care of patients. Methods of treatment will always change but patients' problems never will.

I am not altogether against community care but I hope the community can cope with the mentally ill. The basic needs are tolerance, knowledge and care. It doesn't matter whether these things are given within a hospital or in the community, as long as they are given.'

Edie's mantra of tolerance, knowledge and care is as applicable to our roles as leaders as it is to our life working in a caring profession. We need the self-insight and acceptance to tolerate and understand difference and the views of others, we need to be knowledgeable and informed about the context and environment in which we operate and we need to care for others and ourselves.

As a final closing exercise, try and find some time to write a piece that captures your reflections on this first chapter. Consider those concepts that have meaning for you, in particular those that you connected with in a positive way. And, as importantly, those which you found less helpful. I would suggest that those concepts, models and theories which might have seemed less helpful are often the ones you need to revisit over time.

References

Ashforth, B.E. (2001) *Role Transitions in Organisational Life*. London: Lawrence Erlbaum Associates.

Ballatt, J. and Campling, P. (2011) *Intelligent Kindness: reforming the culture of healthcare*. London: RCPsych Publications.

Beardwell, I. and Holden, L. (1997) *Human Resource Management: a contemporary perspective*. London: Pitman.

Blumer, H. (1969) *Symbolic Interactionism: perspective and method*. Los Angeles, CA: Unversity of California Press.

Dawson, J. (2009) *Does the Experience of Staff Working in the NHS Link to the Patient Experience of Care? An Analysis of Links between the 2007 Acute Trust Inpatient and NHS Staff Surveys*. Birmingham: Institute for Health Services Effectiveness, Aston Business School.

Dawson, J. (2014) Staff satisfaction and organisational performance: evidence from a longitudinal secondary analysis of the NHS staff survey and outcome data. *Health Services and Delivery Research*, 2(1), 336.

Department of Health (2015) *Better Leadership for Tomorrow: NHS leadership review (The Rose Report)*. London: Department of Health.

Ferlie, E. and Geraghty, K.J. (2007) Professionals in public services organisations. In: Ferlie, E., Lynne Jr, L.E. and Pollitt, C. (eds) *The Oxford Handbook of Public Management*. Oxford: Oxford University Press.

Fish, D. and Coles, C. (1998) *Developing Professional Judgement in Healthcare: learning through the critical appreciation of practice*. Oxford: Butterworth Heinemann.

Friedson, E. (1970) *Profession of Medicine: a study of the social dominance: the social structure of medical care*. New York: Harper and Row.

Friedson, E. (1972) *Profession of Medicine: a study of the sociology of applied knowledge*. New York: Dodd, Mead.

Guggenbuhl-Craig, A. (2015) *Power in the Helping Professions*. Thompson, CT: Spring Publications.

Healy, G. and Kraithman, D. (1996) Women in teaching. In: Colgan, F. and Ledwith, S. (eds) *Women in Organisations*. London: Macmillan.

Hede, A. (2007) The shadow group: towards an explanation of interpersonal conflict in work groups. *Journal of Managerial Psychology*, 22(1), 25–39.

Hochschild, A.R. (1983) *The Managed Heart: commercialisation of human feelings*. Berkeley, CA: University of California Press.

Hogg, M.A. and Vaughan, G.M. (2005) *Social Psychology*. Harlow: Prentice Hall.

Katz, D. and Khan, R.L. (1978) The social psychology of organisations. In: Wilson, D.C. and Rosenfeld, R.H. (eds) *Managing Organisations*. London: McGraw-Hill.

Kelly, G.A. (1953) *The Psychology of Personal Constructs*, vols 1 and 2. New York: Norton.

Kline, R. (2014) *The 'Snowy White Peaks' of the NHS*. London: Middlesex University.

Lingard, L., Garwood, S., Schyrer, C.F. and Spafford, M.M. (2003) A certain art of uncertainty: case presentation and the development of professional identity. *Social Science and Medicine*, 56(3), 603–616.

Mead, G.H. (1934) *Mind, Self and Society from the Standpoint of a Social Behaviorist*. Chicago: University of Chicago.

Miller, S., Hagen, R. and Johnson, M. (2002) Divergent identities? Professions, management and gender. *Public Money and Management*, January-March, 25–30.

Pedler, M.J., Burgoyne, J.G. and Boydell, T.H. (2003) *A Manager's Guide to Leadership*. Maidenhead: McGraw-Hill.

Quinn, J.B., Anderson, P. and Finkelstein, S. (1996) Leveraging intellect. *Academy of Management Executive*, 10(3), 7–27.

Strauss, A., Fagerhaugh, S., Suczek, B. and Weiner, C. (1982) Sentimental work in the technological hospital. *Sociology of Heath and Illness*, 4(3), 254–278.

West, M., Dawson, J., Admasachew, L. and Topakas, A. (2011) *NHS Staff Management and Health Service Quality: Results from the NHS Staff Survey and Related Data*. Birmingham: Aston Business School.

Chapter 2 **Presence and personal impact**

Philippa Williams and Jamie Ripman

'*The 360 feedback brought to my awareness that some of how my peer group perceived me wasn't how I wanted to be perceived. I had quite challenging feedback about my style occasionally being patronising. How do I come across? What was it that I do that made somebody think like this?*' (Assistant Director of Nursing)

'*Be the leader you want to be rather than trying to fit. I think the key for me is being authentic to who you are. I've recognised I am a bit quirky, I am a different leader, I'm not going to be your Stepford Wife kind of director of nursing approach. And you've just got to be comfortable with who you are and be the leader you are meant to be.*' (Director of Nursing)

Both these quotes are from participants on the NHS Leadership Academy Senior Operational Leadership programmes. They bring to life a tension that sometimes exists between how we see ourselves and how others see us – our intentions versus our impact on others. This in turn relates to another competing commitment we can feel: between 'being myself' and 'being corporate' or 'being myself' and 'being what is helpful for the situation'. As a nurse or midwife, you will be very conscious of this; focusing on the patient's needs rather than your own can mean managing your feelings about an individual you find annoying or hiding your anxiety in a new situation in order for the patient to feel confident. We touched on this in Chapter 1 and we'll be exploring both these paradoxes in a practical way throughout this chapter; as leaders, what are some of the practical strategies, approaches and behaviours that can help us navigate the competing commitments we will often feel?

How to be a Nurse or Midwife Leader, First Edition.
Edited by David Ashton, Jamie Ripman and Philippa Williams.
© 2017 John Wiley & Sons, Ltd. Published 2017 by John Wiley & Sons, Ltd.

Defining our terms

So what do we mean by 'presence' and 'personal impact'? And why is it an important part of leadership? These are commonly used terms with a variety of meanings for different people. Let's start with *personal impact*. Our simple working definition of personal impact is: '*how we are perceived by others*'. This is not about our intentions; as our first quotation shows, this person didn't intend to be patronising and yet some people perceived her in that way.

How we are perceived can be based on first impressions; what judgements do people make about you when they first meet you? Confident, quiet, powerful, unassuming, shy, nervous, engaging, arrogant? It could also be about the continuing impression you build up over time: 'He doesn't listen. She's very assertive. She can't say boo to a goose. He's verbose. She's friendly' and so on.

Either way, our working hypothesis is that, as leaders, we need to have the impact we intend as far as we possibly can; this is the beginning of our ability to lead and influence others. It also relates directly to our reputation or 'brand'. What makes you distinctive? How do people know what you stand for? It's the beginning of the answer to the provocative question posed by Rob Goffee and Gareth Jones in their book with the same title: 'Why should anyone be led by you?' (2006). Or (attributed to Maya Angelou), 'People may forget what you said, they may forget what you did, but they will never forget how you made them feel'.

Presence is a more slippery word. We talk about people 'having great presence' which is often equated to personal authority or charisma. This is a 'know it when you see it' kind of word. We can all think of people who seem able to get attention when they need it and who draw others towards them. Another perhaps more helpful way of thinking about presence is that it means 'being present' – being in the moment, giving our full attention to what we are doing. This in turn is connected with our ability to attune to our environment, to notice what's going on for us – and what we infer may be going on for others – to listen deeply, and to be agile in how we respond to what we notice. In itself, this is effective. Most of us respond to those who give us their full attention and most of us have a need to know that we have been properly heard.

The Bath Consultancy Group noticed that many of their clients reported that they were struggling to recruit people at senior level because they perceived that many candidates lacked 'gravitas' or 'depth'. In response, the Group spent time researching and finding a way to describe what people look for in leaders. As you can see in Figure 2.1, they articulated this as authority, presence and impact, where presence, as they describe it, is the ability to 'occupy the leadership space in the moment'.

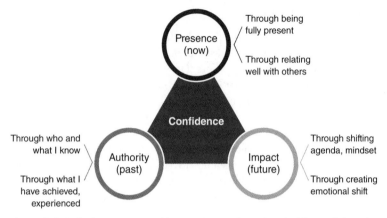

Figure 2.1 Authority, presence and impact. Source: Reproduced with permission of Bath Consultancy Group.

In her book *Presence* (2007), Patsy Rodenburg says:

> '*Here's the problem with the word "presence". Many people believe it is something you have or don't have ... I don't agree: ... you can learn to find your full charisma. All it is, is energy. Present energy – clear, whole and attentive energy.*'

We agree. We think everyone can develop and enhance their personal impact and presence and have spent many years working with people from all types of professions, including nursing and midwifery, to help them do that. The rest of this chapter looks at three key areas, with some practical tools and exercises within each section.

- *Section 1: Developing our personal impact* – in this section we explore how identifying the component parts of our personal impact, and the relationship between those 'parts', can help us be specific about what we need to change or develop in order to create the impact we intend.
- *Section 2: Understanding what's needed for the situation* – this section discusses how our impact is situational; what's appropriate in one context may not be in another. For example, caring for a patient needs a different kind of presence and impact from presenting a paper to the Board or leading a team meeting. We look at some tools and approaches to help us get better at tuning into what different situations require of us and how that can help us adapt our responses appropriately.
- *Section 3: Flexing our style* – we may understand what's needed in these different situations but not be sure how to be different ourselves. This section will look at practical tools and techniques to help us adapt our style.

Section 1: Developing our personal impact

If our impact is about how we're perceived by others, how can we get more control over that? Or, perhaps a more helpful question, what are the areas that we do have control over? Over the past 20 years we have developed an approach that seeks to identify some of the different factors involved in generating those perceptions. This in turn helps us to get really specific about what we can do to align our impact with our intentions more of the time.

Our framework in Figure 2.2 shows an iterative *process* for personal impact development and four key *development areas*. The *process* (the outer circle with arrows) acknowledges the dynamic between the intention we have as leaders and the way others perceive that intention, or our leadership impact. This process encourages leaders to stay curious and interested in where their intention and impact are aligned, and where there is a difference. It also acknowledges the importance of feedback to this process. The first step in developing our impact is to understand how others perceive us; this creates awareness and gives us an indication of what we might need to refine. There are many different ways to gather feedback, for example through the Healthcare Leadership Model 360-degree process, in one-to-ones with your line manager, in supervision. And it can be helpful sometimes to ask for specific feedback, in this case around your personal impact. The following is a practical exercise and suggested approach to help gather feedback.

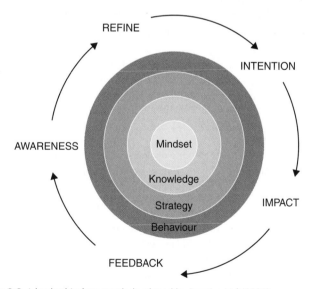

Figure 2.2 A leadership framework developed by Practive Ltd (2003).

BEFORE YOU START

Identify the particular occasion(s) from which you are looking for feedback, e.g. a one-to-one, an informal meeting with colleagues, team meeting, handover meeting, etc.

The next step is to talk with the person giving the feedback and either give them the questionnaire or talk them through it. Let them know the context for the request for feedback, e.g. we are going to be exploring the area of personal impact and it would be helpful to have some personal feedback on the impact that I have on you.

Is there anything else you need to clarify in order that they feel comfortable giving you feedback? For example, will you be sharing their feedback with anyone else?

GATHERING THE FEEDBACK

To the person giving feedback

Firstly, please name the behaviours you noticed in the specific situation that has been identified (e.g. at the meeting that has been identified, when they introduced the purpose of the meeting, what you noticed them do and say was …).

Secondly, describe the impact on you of that behaviour (e.g. 'I felt pleased, uncertain, overwhelmed, excited, relieved, my energy draining away' etc.).

Is there other feedback you would like to give? If so, please give the feedback in a way that describes the impact of the other person's behaviour on you (i.e. rather than saying 'Jane is supportive', say 'I feel supported by Jane when she…').

Making sense of feedback

As you review the feedback, think about these questions:
- How do I feel reading or hearing this feedback?
- What am I surprised about?
- What seems familiar?
- How might I adapt what I tend to do and say in the light of this feedback?
- Do I want to respond to those who have given me feedback?
- What do I want to say? With what intention?

Returning to the framework, the four *development areas* in the middle help us to see where we can make changes to enhance our impact and influence. Some brief definitions follow.
- *Mindset* – by this we mean the beliefs we hold about ourselves, other people and the world, and how these beliefs affect our feelings and thoughts in any

given situation. The notion that it is our *response* to events, rather than the events themselves that affects us is not new: 'There is nothing either good or bad but thinking makes it so' (*Hamlet*, Act II, Sc ii). 'What we are today comes from our thoughts of yesterday, and our present thoughts build our life of tomorrow; our life is the creation of our mind' (Buddha, *Dhammapada*; Mascaro 1973). Advances in neuroscience and psychology confirm that how we perceive the world is partial and that we are prey to cognitive biases and errors in our interpretations of the world around us. 'As we navigate our lives, we normally allow ourselves to be guided by impressions and feelings, and the confidence we have in our intuitive beliefs and preferences is usually justified. But not always. We are often confident even when we are wrong …' (Kahneman, 2011). The more aware we are of how our beliefs and thinking shape our responses, the more we can work with them to give us more choice.

- *Knowledge* – of course, we all need knowledge as leaders. This can be 'technical' knowledge of our professional responsibilities or expertise. It can also be 'soft intelligence': what we know about the individuals and groups with which we interact, about the culture in which we work, about how power and influence are exercised within our organisations.
- *Strategy* – in relation to our personal impact, a strategy might be about how we choose to communicate with others. For example, do we pick up the phone, send an email, walk along the corridor? It could be what we wear to an important meeting, where we sit within that meeting, and how we prepare for it. It could be choosing to ask questions, rather than advocating our own position.
- *Behaviour* – this is about our physical and vocal presence. For example, how we find a strong physical presence where we are centred and grounded, breathing easily, with open body language; where we are using the full range of our voice and our energy is at the appropriate level for the situation; where our body language, gestures, eye contact and non-verbal communication are congruent with the message we are seeking to convey.

All the areas are interlinked and affect each other; for example, if you feel you don't have the *knowledge* you need in a particular situation, you may feel unconfident and think you are not up to the job (*mindset*). This in turn may well come across in your *behaviour* through a tentative voice or closed body language. As we will see later, this can become a bit of a vicious circle; our body language reinforces within us the feelings of anxiety or lack of confidence.

Another way of thinking about these areas is the '*inside-out*' and the '*outside-in*' approach. The 'inside-out' approach is about how by changing our beliefs or thoughts about a situation, we can change the way we behave.

The 'outside-in' approach looks at how changing our behaviour or strategy in a situation can positively affect our mindset and beliefs. To bring this to life, let's take a couple of examples.

Examples of using the framework

Mary was a quietly spoken individual who had a strong belief that 'it's rude to interrupt'. She would sit on the fringe of noisy meetings and find it difficult to make effective contributions. She was feeling frustrated with herself and others. She had good ideas for change on a ward and felt she wasn't being heard and her ideas dismissed. In this case we explored various options for her to make a change.

One option was for her to reframe her *mindset* (making it more acceptable for her to interrupt others). Her belief that 'it's rude to interrupt' went deep. Using some techniques that have evolved from cognitive behavioural therapy (see Chapter 3, 'Things to try'), we explored whether there were any occasions where Mary felt it was acceptable to interrupt. She talked about where there was risk to a patient or a member of staff, or where something really urgent needed communicating. With this in mind, she developed a slightly different thought when entering those situations: 'This is important enough for me to interrupt'. By adding the *strategy* of prefacing the interruption with a helpful phrase such as 'I apologise for interrupting – it feels important before we move on to say that …', she felt that she had given herself permission to interrupt appropriately.

We also thought about what other *strategies* she could use to help her feel more able to contribute. These included talking to her team leader about the possibility of structuring the meetings differently and preparing what she wanted to say in advance (where possible) so that she felt confident she could speak concisely and clearly.

Finally, we looked at how she could use vocal exercises (*behaviour*) to find a more powerful voice when necessary. This was again related to mindset (she came from a family where 'being loud' was frowned upon). Her view of what was 'loud' when she spoke was very different from others. So through using vocal exercises (see last section), she was able to find her voice and through feedback understand that what she felt was 'loud' sounded 'normal' to most people!

Here's another example.

'Throughout my career I have been held back by my fear of delivering presentations and lack of confidence when required to speak in public or to large groups. It is a personal challenge, something I know I must do but definitely not something I relish, and where possible will try to avoid.

I have always envied more extrovert colleagues and charismatic leaders with their ability to communicate complex ideas and goals in a clear, confident and compelling way. This is in stark contrast to my natural preference for introversion ... and a 'quiet leadership' style. I found a practical workshop on improving your physical and vocal presence enlightening. By gaining a better understanding of how the physical effects of fear and stress can negatively affect performance, I have become much more aware of the impact of posture when teaching or public speaking. Simply standing tall and strong, and acting confidently (even if you do not feel it to start with) can facilitate speaking with more confidence and poise. Through learning some very simple voice, breathing and posture exercises and putting them in practice, I have found that my ability to speak with greater confidence when teaching or presenting has improved.' (Specialist Nurse for safeguarding adults in a Clinical Commissioning Group)

This is a good example of an 'outside-in' approach that has helped this leader feel more confident and have a greater impact in situations that she finds personally challenging. Another way to think of this is 'acting as if ...'. As leaders, there will always be times where we need to project something that we aren't necessarily feeling in situations that we find challenging, or when we have conflicting and sometimes contradictory feelings. For example, as a newly qualified nurse you may well be feeling a mixture of excitement and anxiety. It might feel as if one minute you are still a trainee and the next you are expected to take responsibility in a way for which nothing has quite prepared you. The same can apply to someone newly promoted to ward manager and so on. The truth is that, as in many other professions, you will be promoted because you are a good nurse; then you may find yourself leading a team, maybe including people with whom you have previously worked as a peer, or even as a subordinate (remember the role transition ladder and exercise from Chapter 1). At these times, accepting that you are going through a transition is vital whilst acknowledging that you may need to change the way you present yourself.

As one of the nurses on the Leadership Academy Frontline programme said: 'I need to be able to show my team I am confident in my convictions for them to feel they can trust their leader and be behind the decisions I make' (Interim Report on Frontline Leadership Programme, prepared for the Leadership Academy by Hay Group, 2015). So this is not just about feeling confident, it's about projecting it in all situations – even when you are feeling under pressure and less sure of yourself. You could call this the 'performing' aspect of leadership. This is not about pretending to be something you are not, but about being true to your intentions and presenting the part of you that will be most helpful in the situation. And it's important to remember that this may not always feel comfortable. Leadership is not always comfortable and certainly learning new things is not always comfortable! We only have to remember learning to drive to remember those stages of conscious incompetence, followed by conscious competence. The same is true of learning new behaviours, strategies and ways of being with others.

The importance of experimentation and practice

In their article, 'Enacting the true self': towards a theory of embodied authentic leadership', Ladkin and Taylor (2010) ask the question, 'How is it possible to enact a desired leadership self … in never-before-encountered circumstances?'. They reference a study by Ibarra (1999) of young people moving from technical roles to more corporate, leadership positions. Ibarra found that the *least* helpful strategy employed by these young people was when they decided to 'be true to themselves' and she attributed this lack of success 'to their acting in accordance with their feelings of immaturity and inexperience, rather than in accordance with their current situation and possible selves ….'. Those who 'tried out' other ways of behaving were in the long run more successful at finding ways of being that were not experienced as 'fake'. She writes: 'By rehearsing these clumsy, often ineffective, sometimes inauthentic selves they learned more about the limitations and potential of their repertoires and thus began to make decisions about what elements to keep, refine, reject or continue to search for'.

This notion of rehearsal, of experimentation and practice, trying things on for size, is at the heart of how we can develop and refine the impact we have on others.

Section 2: Understanding what's needed for the situation

Which brings us to the next section. How do we understand, prepare for and tune into what's needed in different situations? As we've established, as you move through your career the situations will change and you will need to adapt accordingly. This is a senior nurse from a large acute trust speaking. We'll call her Sarah.

'For me I've been moving into a different arena – a corporate role. I'm having a lot of conversations with Board members and the public as well as my colleagues. It's made me really think about "what do I say in meetings?", "how do I say it?", "how do I hold myself?". Made me take time to think about what I say, what my key points are, recognising sometimes less is more. Giving myself that 20 minutes – who are the different

individuals in the room, where are they going to be coming from, what might be their perspective? It means I'm not so reactive. I'm a bit more cool, calm – I've anticipated it. Where I haven't anticipated it I can ask a few more open questions about why that might be the case.

And there's something about that presence that gives you the confidence – that open body language. It shows I'm open to receiving. I'm not sitting there with my arms crossed looking really worried about what's being said. But also giving myself a few minutes – you don't have to respond immediately, you don't have to react immediately. That open style, going in with confidence even if you're paddling underneath.' (Assistant Director of Nursing)

We can see from this that Sarah has developed *strategies* to deal with this change of context for her – very different from a frontline nursing role or even a senior operational role. She knows she needs to prepare what she wants to say in order to make sure she can get it across succinctly. She also knows how her *behaviour*, specifically her physical presence, has an impact both on others (how they perceive her) and on herself (giving her time to stay calmer and think). She recognises that everyone in that room will have a slightly different perspective, viewpoint, way of thinking. She gives herself time to think about that and then prepares herself so that in the meeting she is best able to notice what is going on and respond accordingly.

Understanding difference

Let's separate these strands out and think first about understanding difference. There are many ways of thinking about how we are different from each other. This includes personal style, culture, age, gender, race, sexuality, learning preferences. We all see the world slightly differently and therefore look for different things. When we think about the gap between intention and impact, this means that part of that gap may well be caused by different expectations or preference on the part of others. For example, a common reason for crossed communication is where there is a difference between how we prefer to receive information and where we focus our attention first. The Myers Briggs Type Indicator® (MBTI®) describes this as the difference between those who have a preference for Sensing (who look first for the detail) and those who have a preference for 'iNtuition' (who look first for the big picture, or the headline). So somebody who prefers Sensing will tend to seek out the facts and detail, will like step-by-step explanations and will prefer down-to-earth, plain language. Somebody with a preference for iNtuition may become bored or impatient with details, and will want to understand the big picture, patterns and relationships, not just the facts (Dunning, 2003).

Let's take an example of how this difference might affect our impact on others. Imagine Mike, a newly qualified nurse, explaining to Jasmine, a patient who is being discharged, what she needs to do to continue with the medication that she has been taking whilst in hospital. Mike patiently starts his explanation from the beginning of the day and talks Jasmine through what she needs to take when. He feels happy that he's done a good job of talking through the detail and, as he is focused on the paperwork to make sure he gets it right, doesn't pick up that Jasmine is looking a bit bemused. So he is surprised when later on he hears that she has complained to the ward sister that Mike is 'really unsympathetic and cold. He didn't look me in the eye and I didn't know why he was telling me all this stuff'.

There's undoubtedly lots going on here, but looking at it through the 'personal impact' lens, we can see that Jasmine has described the impact Mike has had on her: 'He's unsympathetic and cold'. We know that isn't Mike's intention. What has caused the gap? One reason could be that Mike is communicating the detail of the medication to Jasmine in a way that he likes to receive information – calmly, methodically, making sure it's accurate, checking the facts. Unfortunately, this in turn meant that he lost eye contact and that he forgot to give Jasmine the bigger picture: simply that she would need to continue her existing medication for five more days until the follow-up visit to her GP, and that the regime was a little complicated so she would need to follow the instructions. We'll explore these communication gaps more in the chapter on 'getting my message across'. At this moment, though, it's helpful to understand that our differences will affect how others perceive us.

So, given Mike can't control another person's preference in how they receive information, what can he do to make sure that he is better able to tune into Jasmine's needs and then to alter what he does in order to have a different impact? Using our model of impact, we might break it down as follows.

- *Knowledge* – understanding self. If Mike knows that he is focused on detail, and that others aren't, he is more able to check how he approaches these interactions.
- *Strategy* – checking in with Jasmine. What would be most helpful to her in explaining her medication protocols?
- *Behaviour* – eye contact! If we don't look at somebody, it will be difficult to pick up the non-verbal clues.

We've used one particular lens here for thinking about difference. Of course, there are many more. Perhaps one of the most important points here is that in order to have the impact we want, we need to cultivate a mindset and approach of genuine curiosity and interest in those differences. The more we know and are comfortable with ourselves, the more able we are to be interested in others and in exploring how we can work with the glorious diversity around us (Wiseman, 2015).

Preparation

*'Now, I love a party. I do … The problems come just before they start. 'Come as you are'=the original lie. Unless you are Truman Capote or Dorothy Parker – Kanye at a push – never, ever come to a party as you are. **Instead carefully calculate which particular you is required.** As I get older, I have to recalibrate on the doorstep.'* (Eva Wiseman, *The Guardian Magazine*, 19 July 2015)

The emphasis in the above quotation is our own. This is a light-hearted take on preparing 'the particular you' that is required in any given situation. Preparing ourselves for situations is one of the most helpful strategies we know! This is not just about preparing content, although this is of course important; it's about preparing how we want to be in different situations. The importance of thinking ahead comes through strongly in Sarah's narrative. She took on a new corporate role and adapted her behaviour in order to have a different impact in a board setting. She realised that there were different expectations and that she needed to come across as confident and open in order to be listened to and taken seriously.

As a strategy for preparing how you want to be – and be perceived – in specific situations, ask yourself:

• What's my positive intention in this situation?
• What do I already know about the other people involved and their expectations?
• What might I need to do in order to balance effectively my intentions with their expectations?

Responding 'in the moment'

We can see that in order to adjust our impact, it's helpful to understand how others are different, what they might be looking for, and what their expectations are. We can prepare for that and find out as much as we can, but of course we can't prepare for everything. How do we tune in to people and situations effectively in order to be able to respond with the impact we want? This takes us back to the notion of 'presence'; being really present means we notice what is going on, both for us and for others, and this in turn helps us to know how we may need to adapt and flex our style appropriately. It's about giving absolute attention to the other person or people so that they feel 'heard'. Mindfulness is a helpful practice that helps us stay focused on the present moment (see Chapter 3, Mindfulness, for some practical exercises). Connecting with a strong, centred physical presence (see final section of this chapter) also helps. Being present requires us to be open and curious enough to listen deeply, to pick up the signals we are being given by others in order to respond to them. A framework of three 'levels' of listening can help us with this (this framework was used on the Leadership Academy's programme for Senior Operational Leaders).

- *Level 1* – I am thinking about myself. I am preoccupied with what I want, what I am feeling and what I might want to say. In my communicating, I am worrying about what I am saying and what I should say next.
- *Level 2* – I am concentrating on the other person or people. I am interested and intrigued. I am aware of my own judgements and able to put them to one side. I am hearing the values they espouse. My body language is mirroring theirs. I am able to summarise exactly what they have been saying.
- *Level 3* – I am 'super-aware'. I am fully attuned to the other person and aware of my own feelings, judgements and responses. I hear the music behind the words. I notice changes in body movement, voice and energy. I am using my intuition and instincts.

Developing listening skills

These levels are a helpful way of noticing what we pay attention to in any given situation. In which situations do we find it easiest to get to levels 2 and 3 and where do we find ourselves stuck at level 1? Even having these levels in mind can help us to check – where's my attention now?

When asked 'what makes a good leader?', in our experience many people will cite listening as a key quality. In terms of our personal impact, it's not only essential to help us adjust and adapt but in itself, because of the quality of attention it involves, it affects others. And listening well is not always easy, so practising can help us sharpen up our skills and abilities. One way to do this is to separate out the different 'channels' we use to listen to others. So, when I am listening I can pay attention to:

- the words
- the physical signs: posture (open/closed), gestures and movements (foot tapping/hand clenching/passive/active, etc.), eye contact, facial expressions
- the vocal signs: tone, volume, modulation, resonance, depth, congruence with the content and the physical signs
- the impact on me: what reactions am I having? What feelings/thoughts am I having in response? Are these what I would expect or are they surprising? Could these feelings be something I am picking up from the other? What are my hunches, judgements and assumptions? What images do I notice my listening has created? What are the metaphors?

Try this exercise to develop your listening skills.

1 Find a partner who will work with you to develop skills.

2 Each of you, in turn, talks for a few minutes about a dilemma or problem that you would like to solve, that is important to you.

3 As the other person speaks, deliberately 'tune in' to the different channels, one at a time. Start with the body language. What do you notice? How is the body language linked to the words? Then do the same with the tone of voice (close your eyes for a bit if it's easier – having agreed this with your partner!) and finally spend some time noticing how you are affected by what the other person is saying. What are you feeling and thinking about what they are saying? What are your hunches and judgements?

4 Play back to the other person what you have noticed, tuning in to each different channel. Be as specific as you can and, *most importantly,* separate the data you observed from your hunches. For example, 'when you spoke about the new role your voice dropped and you looked away' is <u>data</u>. 'You are anxious about the new job' is your <u>assumption or hunch</u>.

5 Check in with the other person – how did they find you playing back what you had noticed? What impact did this have on them?

6 Swap roles and repeat.

The above exercise and the following ideas are drawn from work we've done with many different groups of people on some of the key principles and skills involved in being attentive to others. From this work it appears that to be a good listener you need to consider technique and awareness/ approach.

In terms of technique:

- be aware of the four 'channels' of listening (see above)
- acknowledge that listening to all four channels in any one moment is impossible, that doing it in any one conversation is difficult and so give yourself sufficient time to prepare
- understand the importance of asking good questions that show you are listening
- check your observations of the data and the assumptions/inferences, e.g. by sharing the observation and testing out the inference
- separate your hunches, judgements and assumptions from the data
- be confident to say what's happening for you, e.g. by disclosing when you have been distracted by your own thoughts.

In terms of your awareness/approach:

- be aware of your own preferences (e.g. Sensing or iNtuitive (MBTI®)) and how this affects the way you listen

- be aware of how your physical and vocal presence may affect others and make changes if necessary
- be able to take a 'helicopter view' in the conversation and notice what is happening as if you were observing
- be able to notice what is happening with your relationships with others in the conversation, and make choices about how to adapt your behaviour in response if necessary.

Listening/tuning in is difficult and requires practice. Fortunately, we are surrounded by opportunities! It doesn't have to be limited to exercises (although these are incredibly helpful); think about all the meetings you go to where you may be able to practise tuning in to a different channel for a while, or noticing where you are placing your attention and how you can shift that.

Embodied leadership

'*I have been trained to communicate and thought that I was quite good at it. Being asked, then, to stand in front of a group and make an impromptu presentation really brought home how other people see me and how easily one's audience can miss the message, simply because of the way I might present myself.*' (Participant on the Frontline Nursing and Midwifery Leadership Programme)

This is one more example of needing to understand and adapt to the situation or different expectations. It has a different focus that leads us into the final section and is about knowing how our *behaviour* can strongly influence how we are perceived. This might be to do with body language, tone of voice, eye contact; human beings are notoriously easily distracted by non-verbal signals. If the non-verbal communication doesn't match with the words, we tend to believe the non-verbal information. So if you are attempting to be inspiring and your vocal delivery is flat and monotonous we will find it difficult to believe you. If somebody is fidgety and doesn't make eye contact, we tend to jump to conclusions about that person, *based on our own beliefs and preferences*: 'She's not confident', 'He's bored', 'She's anxious – or even lying'. One estimate is that more than 60% of social meaning in interpersonal interchange is transmitted non-verbally (Burgoon *et al.*, 1994). Of course, this is a complex area; we can be accurate in our interpretation of others' body language, we can also get it wrong and jump to conclusions. The important point here is that there is a lot of evidence that suggests that we regard the non-verbal cues as more reliable than the words. 'What you do speaks so loudly, I cannot hear what you say' (Ralph Waldo Emmerson, 1876).

Ladkin and Taylor (2010) call this the 'embodied' as well as the 'intentional' aspects of a leader's enactment of their role. This in turn relates back to the first quote of this chapter and the theme of 'being myself' or 'being authentic'. They talk of an assumption in much of the work on authentic leadership that 'one's true self' 'will **automatically be communicated to followers** who will experience the leader as authentic' (our emphasis). They go on to say:

> '... *for the purposes of our argument it is important to point out that it is the leader's body, and the way he or she uses it to express their 'true self' which is the seemingly invisible mechanism through which authenticity is conveyed to others ... We believe recognition of the bodily aspect of leadership is critical to understanding how authentic leadership is perceived.*'

In the first two sections we have looked at how we can shift our *mindset* about a situation to create more chance of responding differently, at expanding our *knowledge* of difference and at some of the *strategies* we can use to help us tune into others and give ourselves the greatest chance of being at our best. In the final part of this chapter, we will explore how we can gain more control over our physical and vocal presence to embody our leadership intentions.

Section 3: Flexing our style when we need to

So, as you will gather, our hypothesis is that there are times when leadership is a 'performing art' – when the situation or context requires behaviours from us that don't fit comfortably with our 'natural' style or our 'typical' way of doing something.

Over the course of running the Nursing and Midwifery Leadership programmes for the NHS Leadership Academy, we heard many examples of where nurses and midwives at all levels were required to 'act into' new ways of doing things because of the requirement of the role or the situation or the people they were trying to influence.

> '*And on my journey towards becoming a Chief Nurse it has made me think about what transition I needed to make from being me now to being a Director. And now my big mantra is: I think like a Director, I speak like a Director, and I act like a Director.*' (Deputy Chief Nurse)

> '*I've been able to recognise what I was doing when I was being effective and feeling good and I'm taking control of my behaviours to repeat these things to ensure I'm acting at my best more of the time. I've found this very empowering and I've recognised that I have the power to take control and that it's my responsibility to do this.*' (Matron)

This has also been our own personal journey. Our original careers were in the performing arts and, in those days, we were adapting and flexing our voice and behaviours to play a character on radio, stage or screen. In our leadership work we are still flexing our behaviours in order to be congruent with our authentic intentions. We are overcoming nerves when standing in front of large groups, changing our vocal and physical energy between different sessions and, sometimes, still getting feedback that our impact hasn't always matched our intentions. This is ongoing work, even for us, and we're supposed to be the experts!

What we know is that there is a part of our training as performers that we still rely on heavily when we need to flex our style. We rely on it every day of our working lives and it has helped us through many high-pressured situations and often enabled us to appear calm, measured and confident when our inner dialogue is arguing strongly that we are imposters.

So, in this final section of this chapter we want to share with you some simple exercises and techniques that we use ourselves and that we have shared with others to help gain a bit more control over our physical and vocal presence when we need to flex our style, manage our nerves or overcome an unhelpful mindset. Depending on your area of clinical expertise, we appreciate that you may be familiar with a lot of what we're about to share. Indeed, some of the exercises below have been adapted and influenced by our work with nurses and midwives.

As you will have read, one of the strands at the heart of our personal impact model is the relationship between our mindset and our behaviours. As performers, we came across this in the form of a simple framework that was developed by an actors' teacher at the Bristol Old Vic Theatre School called Rudi Shelly. It's usually referred to, for obvious reasons, as the mind, body, voice triangle – or the Rudi Shelly diagram of basics (Figure 2.3).

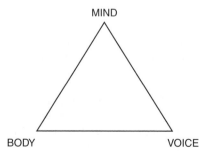

Figure 2.3 Rudi Shelly diagram of basics.

The model is a reminder to performers that the starting point for any change of behaviour can begin in any one of these areas and that by making a start in one area, it will have an effect on another. In reality, performers work on all these areas in the safety of a rehearsal room, experimenting in front of their colleagues with different voices, postures, gestures and character 'intentions' (mindset) to journey towards the creation of a new authentic character.

Whilst this sounds obviously different from the culture that exists in many other working environments (imagine starting your working day with a physical and vocal warm-up in front of your colleagues and patients!), we have found that there are some subtle and practical ways to build up some daily practice and to prepare the body and voice for the rigours and demands of the working day. Because we cover many aspects of mindset preparation elsewhere in this book (working 'inside-out'), we are going to focus the final part of this chapter on some physical and vocal exercises that have helped colleagues to be more congruent with their behaviours and so build up their confidence (working 'outside-in'). After all, your leadership is experienced by others through what you do with the whole of your body, not just what you have prepared in your head. In our experience, with a little extra preparation of our physical and vocal assets we stand the best chance of being confident that we are having the impact we intend, rather than giving a mixed message because our physical or vocal energy is giving a different message to the words we are speaking.

Of course, it's very possible that many of the necessary physical and vocal changes you need to make will happen naturally through your changing thoughts. If you are genuinely more enthusiastic about one idea over another, it is likely that your physical and vocal energy will naturally change to reflect this. The exercises below offer a more technical approach to physical and vocal changes, which can be helpful when old habits and patterns of behaviour are harder to change. Your voice might feel a bit 'stuck' in one place which means that it doesn't change much between expressing something with enthusiasm or with authority. You might notice how you can't control your nerves in certain situations and this has an impact on your breathing and/or rate of speech. You might be naturally softly spoken and you find it hard to raise the volume of your voice to be heard at a team meeting. If so, there are some exercises and techniques that can help. We learnt them as performers and rely on them to this day.

Before we get into the exercises themselves, we'd like to make one important note of explanation and caution. In a book of this length, we have chosen to describe the exercises believing that if you have any physical or vocal condition that means that you can't or shouldn't undertake these exercises, you will take personal responsibility for taking care of yourself. We hope you understand the constraints within which we are writing this. We don't know your body and voice and you do. Please be sensible. We know these exercise can be extremely helpful but we are not recommending them to everyone. Please experiment wisely and within your own limits of safety.

Learning the exercises

As we've indicated, it's very possible that your work and, indeed, even your home environment won't make it easy for you to learn and practise these exercises without being self-conscious. Unfortunately, they can't be done in your head (this is definitely one part of this book that you can't just read to yourself!) and you will have to find a place where you feel comfortable enough to experiment with them. This is a bit like going to the gym with your voice as well as your body; we're going to give specific muscles a bit of a workout while we try to relax others, you'll make some strange noises to help you find your vocal power and then turn that control into everyday speech. The aim is to do these exercises little and often, to build up strength in muscles that may have had less attention recently (like the muscles in your diaphragm) and, ultimately, to create what is sometimes called a muscle memory of how your body and voice need to feel to provide you with a resource that you can easily adapt and flex to different situations.

> 'I feel that my confidence has really improved. Using these breathing and physical techniques I'm able to present cases, issues and discussions at meetings without blushing.' (CCG Assistant Director of Nursing and Quality)

Before you start

Take this book to a place where it will be possible to experiment physically and vocally without feeling self-conscious. The aim is to commit yourself physically and vocally to these exercises and, over time, to learn what feels helpful to you and to turn them into a short routine that you can do anywhere (more of this later). By the way, you may need an office-type or dinner table-type chair and some towels and a pillow to help you get started!

Lying, sitting or standing?

If you are new to this type of work, we strongly recommend that you begin by doing these exercises whilst lying on the floor. It's the easiest and quickest way to create the muscle memory you'll need to develop over time and you'll have the assistance of gravity as well! The ideal position is to lie on the floor with your head on a small pillow or rolled-up towel so that your gaze is directly up at the celling. Without a pillow, your head will fall too far back. The best position for your legs is to put your feet and calves on a chair so that your thighs are at right angles to the floor.

Once you have learnt the exercises in this position, you should repeat them standing and sitting so that you get used to using your voice and body as you do at work.

Getting rid of unhelpful tension

Please take a few moments to release any unhelpful physical tension you might be carrying. Typically, in our daily lives, we build up significant physical tension in our arms, legs, shoulders and neck areas. If you start by working on the floor then take a few minutes to physically relax before doing the exercises below. If you are staying upright, shake out any useless tension. This can include:

- shoulder rolls – forwards and backwards
- shaking out our arms and legs
- easing out the tension in our necks.

The body needs to experience what it feels like to have a powerful constructive tension to support our actions.

Whether lying, sitting or standing, here is a series of exercises which can form the basis of a regular 5–10-minute routine that you can do at home or at various points on your journey into work. Some of these exercises are silent and can be done in the privacy of a bathroom at home or in a toilet cubicle at work. For some of the noisier exercises, you'll have to find a place where you can experiment without feeling self-conscious. On your walk to and from the station, walking the dog, in your car (when stationary) are a few possible options.

START WITH THE BREATH

- Place your hand just above the belt area of your tummy. Over the course of these exercises, we're going to make a strong connection between a physical effort you make here (which we'll call your 'centre') and your voice.
- Start by 'sniffing' in a few short breaths or do one loud 'sniff' in and then breathe out and breathe normally. Notice how your stomach moves out as you sniff in. This tummy movement is caused by the descent of your diaphragm and is the type of diaphragmatic breath you are aiming to maintain and strengthen through the session. Try to keep the upper chest still whilst you use the diaphragm to take in the breath. Repeat this a few times so that you get a good sense of the power of your descending diaphragm (which you will experience through the movement of your tummy).

- Now take in a slower diaphragmatic breath through your nose. Try to repeat the sensation of the diaphragmatic intake of breath and, on the breath out, make the steady and prolonged sound '*shhhh*' (as in 'please be quiet'!). Your aim is to keep the sound going to the end of your breath, without any peaks or troughs in volume.
- Repeat this several times so you get used to this connection between the diaphragmatic effort in your centre and the sounds that you make. This is an essential link that you'll need to maintain throughout the session.

START TO USE THE VOICE

- Continue to take in a diaphragmatic breath through the nose and now, on your breath out, make a loud yawning or sighing sound. Open the back of the throat, keep the tongue flat, drop the jaw and enjoy a loud sigh or yawn. It's first thing in the morning – go for it! *Aaaagghhhhh!* Don't worry about the quality of the sound at this stage; we're trying to create a strong connection between an effort in your centre and the sounds you are making.
- Repeat several times – all the time trying to strengthen the connection between an energy above the belt area and the sounds you are making.
- Using the same technique, now refine the sound so it sounds like a chanted '*ah*'.
- Repeat several times and make sure the sound isn't too 'breathy'. You are aiming to convert as much of the air into sound as possible which will make the voice sound stronger.

PITCH AND RESONANCE

- Now do exactly the same as the previous exercise but close your lips so that you are humming when you breathe out. *Mmmmmmmmmm.*
- Notice where that sound is resonating. It could be anywhere from the upper part of your head to your chest. Where we resonate our voice can have a big impact on how it is perceived. For day-to-day communication it can help to resonate the voice using the resonating spaces at the front of the face.
- Try this as an experiment. Continuing to use the diaphragmatic breath to power the voice, start humming as in the previous exercise.
- Wherever your voice is resonating at first, try to adjust the note of your voice so that the note can help you to bring the voice forward so that you are humming into your lips. It might take you a few attempts but you should start to feel as though your lips are buzzing with the energy of the hum.

- On the next breath, start the hum on your lips and then open them up into the resulting 'ah' sound. *Mmmmmaaaaaaaaaahhhhhhh.* The result should be a slightly brightened vowel sound. Try it a few times more.
- Then try it on a few more vowel sounds and try it on a few different notes to get used to varying the pitch of your voice:
  - *Mmmm .....Ah* as in M<u>a</u>rs
  - *Mmmm .....Eh* as in M<u>e</u>n
  - *Mmmm .....Ee* as in M<u>ee</u>t
  - *Mmmm .....Oh* as in M<u>o</u>le
  - *Mmmm .....Oo* as in M<u>oo</u>n

MOVING FROM CHANTING TO SPEAKING

- By now you should be producing a variety of well-placed, chanted vowel sounds which are energised from your centre by your diaphragmatic breath. You are now going to repeat this technique for the spoken word so the next series of exercises is designed to move you from chanting to speaking.
- You're going to start by chanting the word 'won' or 'one'. In the same way as you chanted the sound *Mmmmaaaahhhh*, you're going to chant the sound *Wuuuuhhhhhh* – it's the beginning of the word 'won'. Use the muscularity of the lips to energise the 'w' at the start of the sound and then support the vowel sound with good energy from your centre. Try it a few more times.
- Then gradually shorten the chant bit by bit until you are making a very short, strong chanted sound, 'wuh'. You should almost feel the kick of your diaphragm muscle as you make this sound.
- Then prepare to use the same technique to speak the word 'won'. Not chanted but spoken. 'Won.' Imagine you are presenting in front of a group and you have this one word to show the power and resonance of your voice. 'One.'
- Now build this into a slow count. *One* (breath in), *Two* (breath in), *Three* (breath in), *Four* (breath in), *Five*.
- Just check you are still feeling a strong connection to the support from your centre. If not, go back a few steps and bring that connection with you as you try again.
- Now build this into a few short sentences and link these words together on one breath: '*One Two Three Four Five*'. Keep the words supported with energy from your centre to the end of the sentence.
- Then try with the days of the week and the months of the year.

By now, you should be feeling that you are using your speaking voice that is initiated by your diaphragmatic breath and then permanently supported by a connection to the energy in your centre.

WARMING UP THE MUSCLES OF ARTICULATION

- Chew some imaginary chewing gum to loosen up your jaw and exercise your lips.
- Triple the size of that gum and keep chewing.
- Press the lips hard together, hold and release.
- To strengthen your tongue, start with it behind your front teeth and roll it back along your hard palate, putting pressure on the palate, and back again.
- Massage the face, especially the jaw, to remove any tension.

PUTTING IT ALL TOGETHER

- Finish your routine with a few tongue-twisters. You may have your own favourites – below are a few of ours. Keep energising your voice from the centre and experiment with different notes and by resonating the voice in different places.
- Create exaggerated enthusiasm by bringing the voice forward.
- Create exaggerated warmth and authority by using more throat and chest resonance.
- Create comedy by using some high notes and lifting the voice into your upper head.
- Here are the tongue-twisters:
  - *Papperty, pepperty, pipperty, popperty, pupperty*
  - *Babberdy, bebberdy, bibberdy, bobberdy, bubberdy*
  - *Tatterty, tetterty, titterty, totterty, tutterty*
  - *Dadderdy, dedderdy, didderdy, dodderdy, dudderdy*
  - *Mammermi, memmermi, mimmermi, mommermi, mummermi*
  - *Red lorry, yellow lorry, red lorry, yellow lorry (repeated)*
  - *Can you imagine an imaginary menagerie manager imagining managing an imaginary menagerie*
  - *She stood upon the balcony, inexplicably mimicking him hiccupping and amicably welcoming him in.*

By using your centre, aim to develop more control of the placing, volume, pitch and pace of your voice, while keeping physically relaxed in the rest of your body. Experiment with nursery rhymes, stories, speeches or poetry. When practising on your own, experiment by exaggerating the range of your voice.

'*I acted up as Chief Nurse at the Board on Tuesday and I knew it was going to be a really difficult meeting and I was expecting several challenging comments and questions. So, I dropped my shoulders, I lowered my voice and I made sure I was calmer and slower in how I spoke so that I wouldn't inject any element of panic and hostility that I felt inside. And it absolutely worked because what would normally have been a complete hammering for an hour turned out to be one question. When people don't see how agitated you feel it diminishes the power that they have over you.*' (Deputy Chief Nurse)

A BREATHING TECHNIQUE TO CALM AND CENTRE THE BREATH

This can be very helpful before giving presentations or challenging meetings if you are starting to feel anxious and particularly if you feel you are getting short of breath.

- Raise an index finger to about 1 ft (30 cm) in front of you and imagine it is a small lit candle.
- Take in a diaphragmatic breath with ease and then breathe out as if you are trying to make the candle's flame gently flicker in the breeze of your breath.
- Your focus should be on the breath out rather than the breath in, which will happen naturally. People often experience a calming effect of this quite quickly.

And finally - power posing

American social psychologist Amy Cuddy has carried out experiments into how our non-verbal expressions of power (i.e. expansive, open, space-occupying postures) affect our own physiology, behaviours, feelings and hormone levels. In particular, she discovered that by adopting body postures associated with power and dominance (imagine that you are showing off that you have just become world champion at the thing you do best) for just two minutes, you can increase your dominance hormone, decrease your stress hormone, increase your appetite for risk, and perform better in interviews and challenging meetings. We've now shared this with many nurses and midwives and have been really encouraged by the results. Take a look at Amy Cuddy's TED talk and give it a go (www.ted.com/talks/amy_cuddy_your_body_language_shapes_who_you_are.html or go to www.ted.com and put Amy Cuddy in the search window) (Cuddy, 2012).

'*The hospital I work at has a state of the art simulation suite and on some study days my team are asked to carry out workplace scenarios. The team is as it would be on shift so, being a senior nurse and nurse in* charge, that was my role. There were also senior consultants, nurses and professors observing. It's all recorded and once you had played out a few scenarios as a team you would watch and critique the video and give feedback to each other. This kind of situation would usually have me wanting to throw myself down the stairs to avoid the whole thing! I couldn't see its value as it was a dummy in the bed and not real!

So I thought I'd give power posing a go before the scenarios commenced, and it changed my life!!! I suddenly became a confident person who engaged fully in the entire day. The feedback I received was amazing and I got so much out of the day. I even had the courage to watch the videos (you could opt out of this part).

I now power pose before any (what I perceive to be) stressful situation. It is such a simple yet valuable tool.' (Senior staff nurse)

References

Burgoon, M., Hunsaker, F.G. and Dawson, E.J. (1994) *Human Communication.* Thousand Oaks, CA: Sage Publications.

Cuddy, A. (2012) *Your body language shapes who you are.* Edinburgh: TED Global 2012.

Dunning, D. (2003) *Introduction to Type® and Communication.* Mountain View, CA: CPP.

Goffee, R. and Jones, G. (2006) *Why should Anyone Be Led by You?* Boston, MA: Harvard Business School Publishing.

Ibarra, H. (1999) Provisional selves: experimenting with image and identity in professional adaptation. *Administrative Science Quarterly,* 44(4), 764–791.

Kahneman, D. (2011) *Thinking Fast and Slow.* New York: Farrar, Straus and Giroux.

Ladkin, D. and Taylor, S. (2010) Enacting the 'true self': towards a theory of embodied authentic leadership. *Leadership Quarterly,* 21(1), 64–74.

Mascaro, J. (1973) *The Dhammapada.* London: Penguin Classics.

Myers Briggs Type Indicator®: www.opp.com

Rodenburg, P. (2007) *Presence. How to use Positive Energy in Every Situation.* London: Michael Joseph.

Wiseman, E. (2015) Getting into the party spirit. *The Eva Wiseman column,* The Guardian Magazine 19 July 2015. London: Guardian News and Media Limited.

Chapter 3 **Surviving and thriving – maintaining resilience**

James Butcher with additional contributions from Nichola Jacob

We think of resilience as 'the capacity to adapt to adversity, while staying mentally, physically, emotionally, and spiritually healthy'. According to Barbara Fredrickson (2009), resilience is not about a detached, dispassionate attitude to the challenges we encounter, but about emotional agility: when we're resilient we worry less ahead of time and rebound more quickly afterwards. We deal with what's in front of us, rather than wasting energy anticipating what might happen, and we revert to an emotional equilibrium without getting caught up in ruminations about what has happened.

But resilience can mean more than simply surviving what life throws at us – human beings have an extraordinary capacity to grow through the experience of adversity, to thrive despite (and even sometimes because of) that adversity. The phenomenon of 'post-traumatic growth' is described by one paper as 'the experience of positive change that occurs as a result of the struggle with highly challenging life circumstances' (Tedeschi and Calhoun, 2004). That struggle can lead someone to think differently about themselves and others close to them, about the emphasis and purpose of their lives, and about the way the world works – a process of reflection and learning.

Fortunately, as the American Psychological Association observes in its online resource '*The Road to Resilience*', the phenomenon of resilience is more ordinary than we might think. A phenomenon called 'hedonic adaptation' (Frederick and Lowenstein, 1999) means that the emotional charge associated with our experiences fades over time. The upside is that we can accommodate to the setbacks we experience – 'time is a great healer', we say to ourselves. So that after a while, an experience like missing out on a promotion we had set our hearts on no longer rankles like it once did. The downside is that we can lose the pleasure and excitement we got from experiences and

How to be a Nurse or Midwife Leader, First Edition.
Edited by David Ashton, Jamie Ripman and Philippa Williams.
© 2017 John Wiley & Sons, Ltd. Published 2017 by John Wiley & Sons, Ltd.

achievements that once filled us with joy. Some of the exercises in Section 3 can help bring back the positive emotional charge to the good things that surround us.

Often resilience is seen as a state of mind – a way to make sense of hardship, to put things in perspective. For example, in their very helpful book on resilience, Karen Reivich and Andrew Shatté say 'it's your thinking style that determines your level of resilience' (Reivich and Shatté, 2002, p. 3). We think it's more than that: we think resilience is about having resources to draw on in challenging times – not just cognitive resources, but emotional, physical and spiritual resources too, an approach in which we focus on ourselves as a whole person. In 'Manage your energy, not your time' (Schwartz and McCarthy, 2007), the authors talk about developing the stamina to deal with demanding jobs, so that instead of running on empty with nothing more to give, we have deep reserves of energy to draw on. Doing so means establishing everyday routines that help develop our whole-person fitness. We expect athletes and performers to practise and prepare, to be fit and ready for their moment of performance – perhaps we can think of ourselves in the same way, taking seriously the demands our jobs place on us, and investing the time and care to prepare ourselves.

In this chapter we look at the ways in which we can strengthen our mental, emotional, spiritual and physical resources, so that we develop that whole-person resilience.

Section 1: Our cognitive selves

'I make sure I'm not accepting things at face value and check out my assumptions by asking questions of the people concerned. This helps me see the problem/situation from different angles and helps keep things in perspective and helps with my decision making.' (Oncology nurse consultant)

The simple idea that the way we think affects the way we feel has a long history. In the second century, Roman Emperor and philosopher Marcus Aurelius wrote to himself in his *Meditations* 'If you are distressed by anything external, the pain is not due to the thing itself but to your own estimate of it; and this you have the power to revoke at any moment'. Today cognitive behavioural therapy tells a very similar story, that the way we feel and act arises from the way we think – how we talk to ourselves about a situation and about our capacity to deal with it. And if we can challenge ourselves to think more realistically and helpfully, and question the validity of our beliefs and assumptions, then we can change how we feel and the choices we give ourselves in how to act.

But is it always helpful to be wrestling with our thoughts, trying to knock them into shape? Another practice with a long pedigree is that of mindfulness, in which we notice, acknowledge and accept whatever thoughts and sensations we are experiencing in the moment – without any intention of changing them. This way we can disentangle ourselves from our thoughts, standing aside from them, and recognising that our identity needn't be tied up in the noisy confusion inside our heads.

In both cases, what changes is not anything in the external world but our relationship to the events we experience – we choose a different relationship, and in so doing can free ourselves from the painful emotions we might have expected to feel. So when we look back on mishaps we can more easily keep things in proportion, and when we look ahead we can face challenging situations with greater equanimity, taking things in our stride.

If this idea appeals to you, here are some things you can try. It may be that these approaches are already very familiar to you, in which case your challenge might be to make your good practice more habitual – see Section 6 for more about making a success of personal change.

Things to try

LOOKING AHEAD

Think about a situation you find stressful. Suppose that's happening next week.
- Write down what goes through your mind – what are you telling yourself about the situation, about how other people will behave, about how you will respond, about the chances of a good outcome? How do you feel as a result?
- How much of what you've written would you say to someone else facing a similar situation? If there is something you wouldn't say to someone else because it would be demoralising, why would you say it to yourself?
- To challenge your way of thinking, you can ask yourself about:
  - *Evidence* – do I have good evidence for what I'm thinking, or am I exaggerating or jumping to conclusions? What's a more realistic view?
  - *Exceptions* – what about counter examples that show things in a different light; what might I have overlooked?
  - *Options* – am I pushing some options out of reach? Have I overlooked some options, and left myself with two equally unpalatable alternatives? Have I restricted myself with self-imposed rules ('I have to … I ought to … I should…')?
  - *Consequences* – am I exaggerating the consequences of doing or not doing something? What's the worst that could happen? How likely is that? What could my contingency plan be? How will this seem in five or ten years' time? Are these my good excuses for not doing anything?

- *Responsibility* – am I taking my share (and no more than my share) of the responsibility?
- *Judgements* – am I being unduly harsh on myself or others? Am I making assumptions about other people's intentions? What's a more compassionate, tentative view to take?
- If you were to change the way you think about that situation, how might you feel as a result?

LOOKING AHEAD (2)

If we want to get into the right frame of mind for a challenging situation we can start to think more positively about the outcome we want, and the resources we already have to help us bring about that outcome:
- Imagine you have had a successful outcome – what happened?
- What did you do to make it successful?
- What have you done already that will help?
- What positive qualities do you bring to this situation?
- When have you been successful before in a similar situation?

LOOKING BACK

When things do go wrong, we can easily let the experience unduly affect how we feel about ourselves, and those negative emotions can then monopolise our attention, so that the experience looms much larger than perhaps its significance warrants. Yet as William James, one of the founding fathers of psychology, observed, 'The art of wisdom is knowing what to overlook'. So we can consciously take a different perspective, and in so doing, feel differently about what's happened.
- *The long view* – how will this all seem in five years' time? These events might seem significant now, but in your memories of this part of your life, how significant a place will they occupy?
- *The detective perspective* – what are the facts, rather than your interpretation of them? If you strip out your assumptions and judgements, what are the facts left behind?
- *Turning the tables* – what would you say to someone else in a similar situation? Can you coach and encourage yourself in the way you would someone else?
- *A learning lens* – what can you learn from what has happened, lessons that you take with you in preparation for similar situations in the future?

MINDFULNESS

'I decided to take a bit of a leap of faith and at my last team meeting we practised some mindfulness. I was surprised and really encouraged by the positive response I received. They said it really helped and are keen to continue the practice.' (Quality improvement lead)

Jon Kabat-Zin, who has done so much to bring the practice of mindfulness to a Western, secular audience, describes mindfulness as 'paying attention in a particular way: on purpose, in the present moment, non-judgementally' (Kabat-Zinn, 1994). Instead of reframing our thoughts, we step aside from them for a while, to let our thoughts be what they are and let them pass on by. There are plenty of books, tapes and apps to help you practise mindfulness; here are some simple exercises.

Breathing

The seven-eleven technique is to breathe in for a count of seven, then breathe out for a count of eleven. As you breathe you should feel movement in your abdomen: when you breathe in your diaphragm flattens to create a larger space for your lungs; as a result, your stomach will move outwards, then back in as you breathe out. Let your attention stay focused on those movements, and on the sensation of air passing in through your nose and out through your mouth.

Scanning

Whether sitting or lying down, close your eyes, and let your attention very gradually scan through your body, from the tips of your toes to the top of your head. For each area of your body, notice any physical sensations, perhaps of tension or discomfort, or the sensation of your body against a chair, or clothes against your body.

Mindful moments

We can also create mindful moments for ourselves. These days it's easy to occupy any spare moment checking our phones for emails, Facebook updates and tweets. What if we were to spend the few minutes we have waiting for a train just being in the moment, noticing what's happening around us and within us, simply connecting ourselves to the present moment rather than distracting ourselves away from it? Building in short breaks at work, for just a few minutes, can give you the chance to reflect and take stock, and refresh your attention.

These practices can help us think more realistically and helpfully about the challenges we face, and about difficult times we've been through, helping us maintain a more robust emotional state. As the 14th-century Persian poet Hafez said: 'What we speak becomes the house we live in' – something that applies to the way we speak to ourselves as much as to others. Can we be as encouraging and supportive of ourselves as we would be of others?

Section 2: Our emotional selves

> ' I have just started a new job and one of things I'm really concentrating on is building new relationships and identifying where my support will come from. I wouldn't have done this a while ago but have recognised how important this is for me and my ability to stay resilient.' (Quality improvement lead)

A simple way to think about emotions is as a mechanism for orienting us towards things that are beneficial to us and away from things that might harm us. As neuroscientist Antonio Damasio puts it, 'All emotions have some kind of regulatory role to play ... their role is to assist the organism in maintaining life' (Damasio, 1999). We can think of emotions as 'lights on the dashboard' giving us information about how we need to respond to something happening in our environment. According to Cacioppo *et al.* (1999), 'affect directs attention, guides decision making, stimulates learning, and triggers behaviour' (p. 840). So all emotions are useful and adaptive, whether positive or negative.

Like any control system, this one has its faults. We can feel emotions like anxiety and guilt when we have no cause to – our emotions are firing unnecessarily. And then there are times when we suppress an emotion, ignoring the lights flashing on our dashboard. We might think we 'shouldn't' feel a certain way – we shouldn't get angry so we get upset instead, or we shouldn't be anxious, so we get irritable. As Aristotle said, 'Anybody can become angry – that is easy, but to be angry with the right person and to the right degree and at the right time and for the right purpose, and in the right way – that is not within everybody's power and is not easy'.

We can also think about our internal 'prevailing weather' – is the balance more positive or negative? When we think about our typical day, are we more upbeat or downbeat? Researchers like Alice Isen and Barbara Fredrickson have suggested that there is a value to positive emotions beyond their signalling role. For example, it seems that if we experience more positive emotions, we can then recover more readily from stressful situations – for example, blood pressure returns to normal more quickly after giving a stressful presentation

(Fredrickson, 2003). Fredrickson argues that positive emotions also have a longer term, developmental effect that can 'transform people for the better, making them more optimistic, resilient and socially connected' (ibid.).

This is not about trying to exclude negative emotions, but to get to a reasonable balance. Part of the reason we can end up feeling a disproportionate amount of negative emotion is that we find it easy to overlook good things in our lives, to take them for granted. The psychologist Roy Baumeister and his colleagues wrote a paper entitled 'Bad is stronger than good' (Baumeister *et al.*, 2001) which collects evidence that negative stimuli have a greater impact on us than do positive stimuli; for example, we feel the loss of a sum of money more keenly than we do gaining the same amount.

And we seem to process negative information more thoroughly, and give it greater weight than we do positive information. Our cognitive system has evolved to be wired for alarm more than satisfaction; this keeps us on our toes, alert to danger and disadvantage, and avoiding any kind of complacency that the good things we have are enough. In an unreliable world of shortage, the latter tendency keeps us motivated to keep looking for what we need to stay healthy; in the world of plenty in which most of us now live, we can find it hard ever to be satisfied. The challenge for us is neatly captured in the title of Timothy Miller's book, *How to Want What You Have* (Miller, 1995).

So if we want to change our internal weather, what are some practical things we can do?

Things to try

THREE GOOD THINGS

It's easy on our journey home from work to ruminate on our frustrations from the day – things we left undone or did unsatisfactorily, annoying encounters with colleagues and patients, run-ins with authority figures, wrestles with irritating bureaucracy. It's as if we allow those moments to eclipse all the good, satisfying things that happened, and we can end up in an unnecessarily downbeat mood.

Instead, on your journey home, or at the end of the day, think about three good things from your day.

- *Something to savour* – an experience you enjoyed, something out of the ordinary or something as simple as a few minutes fresh air in the sunshine during a break, or a conversation with colleagues over coffee. Bring the experience to mind as vividly as you can, savouring the details of what happened and the emotions you felt.

- *Something you're grateful for* – something in your life that you value and appreciate, thinking about home and family, friends, work, leisure, health and wellbeing, resources and experiences.
- *Something you want to give yourself a pat on the back for* – something you did that made a positive difference at home or work.

If you can, write your reflections down, to create a store of encouraging good things that you can keep returning to. If you live with someone else, this is an exercise you can do together – sharing your responses can be illuminating.

MANAGING IN THE MOMENT

If we are overtaken by an unexpectedly strong emotional reaction, how can we regain our equilibrium? If you're prone to those kind of reactions it can help to practise spotting the first signs of an emotion building up – the sooner you intervene, the easier it will be to do something that interrupts the cycle.

Breathing

The seven-eleven breathing technique described earlier is something you can do any time, anywhere to steady and calm yourself, and regain your composure.

Movement

Moving physically – changing posture or walking somewhere, even just across the room to get a glass of water – can break the cycle of a strong emotion building up.

On the receiving end

If you're on the receiving end of someone else's strong emotional outbursts, it can help to imagine their words flying over your shoulder, perhaps hitting the wall behind you – while you can notice the words as they hurtle past, without feeling you're the target of them.

It can also help to remember that someone can't be angry forever (even if sometimes it seems that way) – emotions tend to build up and then die down, unless we help stoke them up again. Listening and acknowledging what someone else is feeling can help defuse their emotional response. As Steven Covey reminds us: 'seek first to understand before being understood' (Covey, 1989).

As well as these personal reflections, we can also be thinking about where we get support from. Who are the people we can turn to and rely on for a listening ear and helpful advice? If you're the kind of person who's always there for others, always ready to make time to listen, are you as good at getting the support you need for yourself?

The exercises in this section can help us to change the balance of the emotions we experience, to bring more positive emotions to our lives; doing so can help both in the moment and in building the psychological resources needed for resilience.

Section 3: Our spiritual selves

For some, their spiritual life is about their religious faith. For others, it's about the meaning and purpose they create in their lives, and the values they seek to live by. The more we live in alignment with our values and purpose, the more energised we're likely to be. When we compromise on our values we're likely to experience 'cognitive dissonance', the uncomfortable feeling that comes from a contradiction between our beliefs and our actions. As we can't change what we've done, we tend to erode our beliefs instead – and we risk giving up on what matters to us.

Bill George encourages leaders to identify their 'true north' – their motivations, values and sense of purpose, the end to which their leadership is the means (George, 2004). The more we have our values and purpose clearly in mind, the easier it is to make difficult decisions and live with the consequences. And it's clearer where we should draw our 'lines in the sand' – the boundaries between what we'll accept and what we won't.

We often talk about juggling the many different responsibilities we have. To extend James Patterson's (2001) metaphor, we can imagine that some of the balls we're juggling are made of rubber – if we drop them they'll bounce back. Others are made of wood – if we drop them they'll lie on the floor waiting for us to retrieve them later. And finally, some are made of glass – if we drop them they'll shatter. Being clear about our values and purpose will help us highlight the precious, irreplaceable things in our lives.

Things to try

INTENTION FOR THE DAY

In the morning, as you start the day, tell yourself your intention for the day. What's the impact you want to have on others? What's the difference you want to make? Which of your values do you want to be most conscious of today?

CLARIFYING MY VALUES

Reflect on the list of words below: which 10 do you think best describe your values? If the words aren't quite right, or something's missing, just add your own version.

Achievement	Relationships	Variety	Nature	Status	Integrity
Change	Excellence	Wealth	Competition	Reputation	Friendship
Service	Honesty	Knowledge	Serenity	Contribution	Loyalty
Advancement	Freedom	Novelty	Adventure	Competence	Community
Quality	Helping	Affection	Leadership	Arts	Excitement
Authority	Faith	Harmony	Responsibility	Family	Development
Growth	Independence	Collaboration	Privacy	Recognition	Influencing
Diversity	Justice	Altruism	Fitness	Improvement	Fairness
Reliability	Hard work	Legacy	Discipline	Humility	Generosity
Boldness	Love	Diligence	Joy	Ambition	Fun

Of the 10 words you've chosen, which three are most central to who you are? Thinking about those three words, reflect on the following questions (by yourself or in conversation with someone else).

- What do these three values mean to you?
- Where are these values evident in your life?
- When have they been compromised?
- What could you be doing more of, less of, or differently to live your values more consistently?

Finally, imagine someone following you around for a few days, observing your behaviour and the choices you make – how good a guess could they make about the values you've just articulated?

We asked some nursing and midwifery colleagues what they had found helpful in this area and here are some things they do.

- I give myself time to reflect and think about what's important.
- I play music.
- I think about the greater good.
- I know I make a difference to others.
- I find people to laugh with.
- I reflect and evaluate and think of the nature around me.
- I walk the dog in the early morning.
- I keep connected with my faith and community.
- My sister sends me a daily affirmation on WhatsApp.

Section 4: Our physical selves

It's easy to overlook the fact that our psychology lives in our biology. As we get older, our lives can get more complex and demanding – perhaps we start a family, get promoted, take on caring responsibilities. At the same time, it can feel as if the energy we had 10 years ago isn't quite as readily available – so it becomes ever more important to look after ourselves physically, and think about our diet, our exercise routines and our patterns of sleep. Part of being resilient is having the physical stamina to cope with a demanding job – and if we want to feel positive, confident and resourceful it helps to feel physically buoyant too. Without paying attention to your physical wellbeing, the exercises in the previous section that are intended to help you look after yourself emotionally may not have the impact you'd hope.

While the advice about living healthily is probably well known to you, here is a reminder.

Exercise

At the time of writing, NHS Choices (www.nhs.uk) recommends 150 minutes of exercise a week, with a mixture of aerobic activity and muscle strengthening activity. The site has lots of advice on fitness and flexibility exercise routines, including the 'Couch to 5k' running training programme. Even without a formal exercise programme, there can be lots of opportunities during a day to walk a little more than you usually do – for example, taking the stairs rather than the lift or escalator, getting off the bus a stop earlier, parking a little way from your destination.

Diet

NHS Choices also has advice on a balanced diet, illustrated by the 'Eat Well' plate, showing the recommended proportion of different food groups.

As you would expect, the advice is to eat more fruit, vegetables and fish, and to eat less sugar, salt and saturated fat.

Sleep

Sleep seems to play an important role in sorting and connecting memories, in learning and in forgetting (letting go of memories rather than storing them). The advice is to create a routine around going to bed, so that you start to create a habit of sleep. It can help to avoid caffeine, sugar and alcohol in the hour or so before you go to bed. And it's a good idea to avoid screens in that last hour of the day, and for your bedroom to be softly lit.

Again, we asked colleagues what they had tried that had helped and here are some of their examples.

- I get off the tube one stop early and walk.
- I practise the 'Amy Cuddy' power poses (see Chapter 2).
- I cycle to work and make exercise part of my working day.
- I knit to relax.
- I play with my child as if I'm a three year old.
- I take a lunch break as a minimum three times a week.

Section 5: The challenge of change

We expect that much of this chapter will be familiar to you – the benefits of mindfulness, exercise and so on are discussed regularly in the media. And yet we often experience that uncomfortable gap between knowledge and action, and might ask ourselves, 'why is it hard to do the obvious thing?'. Simply knowing the good advice probably won't be enough for us to adopt different, healthier routines. In this section we look at the conditions necessary for making a success of personal change.

Because you're worth it

The place to start might be our relationship with ourselves. The Buddha said, 'You, yourself, as much as anybody in the entire universe, deserve your love and affection'. But do we believe that? Transactional Analysis uses the deceptively simple language of 'I'm OK, You're OK' to describe a healthy relationship with ourselves and others (Stewart and Joines, 1987). When we can say 'I'm OK', we value ourselves and treat ourselves with compassion and respect. And if we do so, we're more likely to commit to looking after ourselves physically and emotionally, and to have kinder judgements of ourselves.

If you find yourself saying things like 'After all, I'm only a nurse' then it's likely that you've slipped into an 'I'm Not OK' position, where you undervalue yourself and your capacity to influence the world around you. One way to think about that capacity is through Peter Hawkins's model of Authority, Presence and Impact (Hawkins, 2011) that we looked at in the last chapter.

• Your *authority* is about the experience, expertise and achievements that you bring to a situation. You might find yourself downplaying your expertise or overlooking experience you assume might not be relevant. Can you give yourself an honest account of what gives you authority? Do you take yourself seriously, in the way you expect others to?

• Your *presence* is about your ability to be fully in the moment, your attention focused on the people in front of you. People often say of those seen as having great presence, 'It was as if I was the only person in the room'. When you're fully present, you'll notice the subtle shifts in how the other person is communicating – tracking those shifts will help you keep in rapport with them. If you tend to get distracted, your attention fragmented, you might think you can disguise it – the likelihood is that others will notice and feel that disconnection.

• Your *impact* is about your ability to utilise your authority and presence in making a shift in what's happening in front of you. This might be a *cognitive* shift, as you help others to see things in a new light, an *emotional* shift as you help change the climate of a conversation, or a *motivational* shift, as you help to crystallise the commitment of others to action.

Our beliefs about change

The second area to look at is our belief about our capacity to change. In Transactional Analysis the 'discount matrix' describes the ways in which we recognise or discount the existence of a problem and our capacity to deal with it (Stewart and Joines, 1987).

Level 1: discounting the existence of a problem

At this level, we're simply unaware that our behaviour or the impact of a situation amounts to a pattern – we don't notice how tired we are, or we're oblivious to the impact we have on others, or a pattern in our behaviour isn't salient for us. What helps at this level is a habit of seeking feedback from others, of being open to that feedback, and to checking in with ourselves, with scrutiny and honesty.

Level 2: discounting the significance of a problem

At this level, we're aware of an issue, we just don't take it as seriously as we should. For example, faced with the cognitive dissonance between everything we hear about the dangers of smoking and the fact that we smoke, we might discount the information and its relevance to us, and remember instead an uncle who smoked 60 a day and lived to a ripe old age. Or we might be prone to emotional outbursts but tell ourselves that we've always worn our heart on our sleeve, or we feel wiped out at the end of the day but tell ourselves it's 'par for the course'. The 'confirmation bias' means that we're likely to notice information that supports our position and overlook data that's inconvenient to our way of thinking.

At this level we need to challenge our own confirmation bias by looking for evidence that runs counter to our preconceptions, looking for examples that could challenge our settled view of how things stand.

Level 3: discounting the possibility of change

Carol Dweck describes two mindsets: a 'fixed' mindset in which we think of personal strengths and abilities like we would our height – something we can do little to change, and a 'growth' mindset in which we think of our capabilities as more like physical strength, something we can increase through exercise and practice (Dweck, 2006). If we're to learn new ways of thinking, feeling and acting, then clearly we need to believe that such an enterprise is possible, that people have the capacity to change.

At this level, if we have a fixed mindset, we might accept that an issue exists and is serious but believe that change is unlikely – the issue is just something to be lived with. To counter this, we can look for examples of people who have made changes in this area of their lives, role models for the possibility of change.

Level 4: discounting the possibility that we can change

We might believe that on the whole it's possible to get fitter or calmer or achieve better work–life balance, whilst believing that it's not possible for *us*. The psychologist Albert Bandura coined the term 'self-efficacy' – the belief that we can do the things we set out to do: 'Yes we can' as Barack Obama (and Bob the Builder) encourage us to think (Bandura, 1982). Without that belief, we're unlikely to persist with (or even start) efforts to change.

At this level, we accept that change is possible, for others perhaps, but not for us. To counter this we can reflect on all the experiences we have had of changing and developing, examples big and small that show our capacity for growth. We can develop a habit of noticing and celebrating small shifts in our behaviour or in how we think and feel.

So for us to be capable of change, we first need to recognise that a problem exists. As we explored in Chapter 2, feedback from others can help develop our self-awareness, as can mindfulness, which helps us tune into our bodies, hearts and minds, allowing aspects of our internal experience that we had overlooked to come into our attention. We then need to take what we become aware of seriously – to place due value on the impact we have on others, and to value ourselves sufficiently that we recognise the effect that our experiences have on our health and wellbeing. And finally we need to become more alert to the evidence of change in ourselves and others.

Healthy habits

We can think about personal change as a process of developing new habits, of embedding new patterns of behaviour in our daily routines. We don't generally deliberate about whether or not to brush our teeth at night – the behaviour is triggered by our routine at the end of the day and we don't need to think too much about it or summon up any great willpower to get on and do it. For many of us, willpower is not a very effective way to regulate our behaviour, and it consumes a lot of mental energy. So the more we can automate healthy behaviours and establish them as habits, the easier it will be to maintain those behaviours.

According to Charles Duhigg (2012), habits consist of three elements – a cue, a routine and a reward. The cue is some aspect of our environment or our daily life that prompts a behaviour. For example, we might always associate a coffee break with an opportunity for a sweet treat, or the dog waiting restlessly by the back door with going out for a stroll. There is evidence to suggest that far more of our behaviour than we suspect is prompted by environmental cues, rather than deliberate choice (Wilson, 2002).

The second element – the routine – is a new behaviour we want to establish, or an existing behaviour we want to stop. In the latter case, it can help to think about what we want to do *instead*, to have a new behaviour to replace what it is we want to stop doing.

The final element is the reward. For us to establish a new pattern of behaviour, we need to experience a benefit that reinforces the behaviour. We need to be able to connect the behaviour to something that matters to us so that it becomes something we *want* to do, rather than something we feel we *ought* to do. If we're going to embark on a fitness programme or start practising meditation, what will that bring us? What's the benefit, and why does it matter to us? And if we imagine ourselves having succeeded in our endeavours, how do we feel? Excited or indifferent? That emotional response – albeit to an imaginary success – will be a clue as to whether what we're planning matters enough for us to persist with it.

Social support

In his article 'The human moment at work', Edward Hallowell (1999) says: 'Human beings are remarkably resilient. They can deal with almost anything as long as they do not become isolated'. So part of developing resilience is to be able to reach out to others and ask for support and help. When people start to share honestly with others about their frustrations and anxieties, a very common response is 'It's such a relief to find that others feel the same way I do – that I'm not the only one'. When we set out to make changes to the way we live, it can be a great help to know that someone else is concerned for us, encouraging us – and waiting to hear how we get on.

Continuing to learn

As Aimee Mullins says in her TED talk: 'Adversity is just change we haven't adapted ourselves to yet'. We can adapt through reflecting on our experiences and learning from them. That can simply involve taking time out to jot down our thoughts in a journal, and making that process of reflection a habit. Here are some questions that might help prompt your thoughts as you reflect on something that's happened.

• What did I say and do?
• What was I saying to myself?
• What was I feeling?
• What was my intention in the situation?
• How well did my impact match that intention?
• What was surprising about what happened?
• What was familiar?
• Is the way I responded part of a pattern that I've noticed in myself?
• What makes this event matter to me?
• What am I pleased about in how I responded?
• What helped me?
• What hindered me?
• What would I do differently next time?

Some people prefer to reflect privately, others in conversation with somebody else who can help generate fresh perspectives. If you keep a journal you can review it from time to time and see what themes you notice in the different entries, and ask yourself: what's consistent and what's changing?

In summary, making a success of change is partly to do with how we think about ourselves, and about the possibility of change, and partly about our ability to practise new behaviours and persist until we create new habits.

Section 6: Leading resilient teams

Imagine that you're walking along a beach on a wild and windy day. As you look out at the turbulent sea you realise to your horror that there's a swimmer out there clearly in difficulties. Before you can reach for your phone to call for help, you hear the sound of a helicopter flying low overhead, and then you watch as someone is winched down to the waves. They strap the swimmer into a harness, and the two figures are hauled up to safety. Inside the helicopter, the swimmer is being treated by a paramedic. There's a psychologist talking about resilience, and a swimming coach explaining the best techniques for stormy seas. And then from the beach you watch as the swimmer is lowered back down into the waves.

Ridiculous of course, but perhaps a reasonable metaphor for the way in which we can focus all our attention and expectation on individuals and their strengths and weaknesses, and overlook the culture in which those individuals work. So far this chapter has been about you as a leader and how you can strengthen your own resilience. Another aspect is how you lead resilient teams – how do you create the conditions in which others can be resilient?

A straightforward way to think about culture is the behaviours and processes of a team or organisation, and the shared values from which they derive (Hofstede *et al.*, 1990). Leaders are particularly influential in creating and reinforcing cultural norms – sometimes consciously, sometimes unwittingly. In a way, the culture of your team is a reflection of your leadership style. Supposing a new joiner were to ask a long-serving colleague for a real and honest induction after the official one – 'What kind of support do we get?' they might ask. 'Is it OK to ask for help if it all gets too much?' What would that kind of conversation tell you about the norms in your team – not the explicit norms, but life in your team as it's lived.

Connected to the team's culture is its emotional climate. A process called 'emotional contagion' (Hatfield *et al.*, 1994) means that we can be very influenced by the emotional state of others. And leaders are particularly contagious. So taking care of your emotional wellbeing is important not just for you but for the wellbeing of your team too.

Recent research by this author suggests that organisational cultures that help people thrive will be ones that provide the right psychological 'nutrients' – factors that satisfy fundamental psychological needs. Let's take a look at what those psychological nutrients are, and see what questions we might ask ourselves as leaders seeking to develop resilient teams.

Autonomy

Feeling we can control what happens to us is a highly significant contributor to our wellbeing, both mental and physical. In a famous experiment in the 1970s, Langer and Rodin (1976) worked with a nursing home and arranged for residents on two different floors of the home to be given different degrees of autonomy. For example, on one floor, residents were given pot plants to look after, while in the other staff took on the responsibility. The first group of residents were given a choice about visiting arrangements, while on the other floor all that was taken care of by staff. The researchers found that the residents who were given greater control over their lives became more active and alert, had a greater sense of wellbeing, and even lived longer.

When we feel we have little control or influence over our circumstances, we can start to exhibit 'learned helplessness' (Seligman, 1991) – a state where we no longer try to make a difference to what's happening because we have learned that there's little point. Models of organisational change often refer to those who 'resist' or 'block' change – but is that attitude a consequence of the personality of those individuals or a reaction to the culture in which they find themselves?

> How do you ensure that those you manage feel trusted to use their own judgement and initiative where possible, rather than always having to defer to set procedures or the authority of others?
> What would they say about you in this regard?

Belonging

According to Baumeister and Leary (1995), the need to belong is the most fundamental psychological need of all, even 'one of the most far-reaching and integrative constructs currently available to understand human nature' (p. 522), so that much of our behaviour is directed at finding a sense of belonging.

At a simple level, do we feel we're among friends at work? For Buckingham and Clifton (2007), having 'a best friend' at work is one of 12 indicators of a productive organisational culture.

Part of belonging is to recognise ourselves in others, to see people like ourselves in our team and organisation. How many faces like mine do I see around me? How many others are there who share my ethnic background or faith, my experience of disability, or who have a similar sexuality?

> Do those you manage feel that they have a secure place in a team, that they are valued and included, and can count on the support of colleagues? Have a look at your organisation's NHS Staff Survey results, which will give you an indication of how included people feel in your organisation. At a national level there is still much to do, as the national NHS Staff Survey clearly identifies that some colleagues do not feel included.

Meaning and purpose

One way to think about leadership is helping others to 'keep their eyes on the hills and their feet on the path'. We might be good at efficiently managing the day-to-day activities of the team, but do we help them see the larger purpose to which their efforts are contributing? And can people see their own values reflected in the values of the organisation, or do they feel at odds with its ethos? There's evidence that employees who feel that their own values are congruent with the values of the organisation tend to feel more engaged (Bono and Judge, 2003).

Research into 'post-traumatic growth' – the phenomenon of people bouncing back from adversity stronger than before – suggests that an important part of resilience is the capacity to find meaning and sense in what happens to us (Nolen-Hoeksema and Davis, 2004). In *Man's Search for Meaning*, Viktor Frankl describes his experiences in Auschwitz, and says 'striving to find a meaning in one's life is the primary motivational force in man' (Frankl, 1946/2004, p. 104). Survival in the concentration camps about which he wrote was most helped by a sense of meaning, a task or mission beyond the desperate constraints of the present moment.

> To what extent is there a fit between people's personal values and the values of the organisation? How can you ensure that others feel, even more, that their talents and efforts are contributing to something that counts?

Challenge and achievement

We develop and grow through being tested and challenged, having our abilities stretched, and feeling that we are operating on our learning edge. The kind of personal investment required of us when work is challenging is one of the characteristics of employee engagement (Kahn, 1990).

When we successfully work through a challenge there's the satisfaction of both achieving a goal and mastering the skills to do so. If we see that things never seem to come to fruition, that 'task and finish' groups never quite finish and initiatives often peter out, then we're less likely to feel that sense of 'self-efficacy' referred to earlier, the confidence that we can do the things we set out to do.

> To what extent are people you lead able to get the satisfaction from attaining an outcome and mastering the skills required to accomplish it? How might you offer a level of challenge that is stretching without becoming stressful?

Clarity

It helps us to be clear how our organisation works, and what's expected of us, so that we know how best to invest our time and energy. Having that clarity about expectations is an important contributor to employee engagement (Christian *et al.*, 2011).

Perhaps some of what we describe as 'complexity' in organisational life is actually just muddle; sometimes organisations can mistake complication for sophistication. As Einstein said, 'Any intelligent fool can make things bigger and more complicated ... It takes a touch of genius and a lot of courage to move in the opposite direction'.

Another aspect of clarity is knowing what the future holds for the organisation and our place within it. This section has examined how fundamental psychological needs can be satisfied – or not – by the experience we have of work. But work is also the way we satisfy more basic needs – our ability to provide for ourselves and our families. So when the organisation's future is uncertain it can leave us feeling anxious about the things that matter most to us.

At times of organisational upheaval, we may not be able to give clarity about an endpoint – but can we offer some clarity at least about the process by which we'll get there?

How clear are the people you lead about who is responsible for what, and what the organisation's expectations are of them? How do you know this? How can you help them understand more what the future holds for patients, their team and the organisation?

In summary, as leaders we can contribute to the resilience of those we lead through creating the kind of team culture that allows team members to thrive. To do so, we need to make sure that the psychological factors that contribute to people's wellbeing are present in the teams we lead.

References

Bandura, A. (1982) Self-efficacy mechanism in human agency. *American Psychologist*, 37(2), 122–147.

Baumeister, R.F., & Leary, M.R. (1995) The need to belong: desire for interpersonal attachments as a fundamental human motivation. *Psychological Bulletin*, 117(3), 497–529.

Baumeister, R.F., Bratslavsky, E., Finkenauer, C. and Vohs, K.D. (2001) Bad is stronger than good. *Review of General Psychology*, 5(4), 323–370.

Bono, J.E. and Judge, T.A. (2003) Self-concordance at work: toward understanding the motivational effects of transformational leaders. *Academy of Management Journal*, 46(5), 554–571.

Buckingham, M. and Clifton, D. (2007) *Now, Discover Your Strengths*. London: Bloomsbury.

Cacioppo, J.T., Gardner, W.L. and Bernston, G.G. (1999) The affect system has parallel and integrative processing components: form follows function. *Journal of Personality and Social Psychology*, 76(5), 839–855.

Christian, M.S., Garza, A.S. and Slaughter, J.E. (2011) Work engagement: a quantitative review and test of its relations with task and contextual performance. *Personnel Psychology*, 64(1), 89–136.

Covey, S. (1989) *Seven Habits of Highly Effective People*. New York: Simon and Schuster.

Damasio, A. (1999) *The Feeling of What Happens: body and emotion in the making of consciousness*. Fort Worth, TX: Harcourt College Publishers.

Duhigg, C. (2012) *The Power of Habit: why we do what we do in life and business*. New York: Random House.

Dweck, C. (2006) *Mindset: the new psychology of success*. New York: Ballantine Books.

Frankl, V. (1946/2004) *Man's Search for Meaning*. London: Random House.

Frederick, S. and Loewenstein, G. (1999) Hedonic adaptation. In: Kahneman, D., Diener, E. and Schwarz, N. (eds) *Well-Being: the foundations of hedonic psychology* New York: Russell Sage Foundation, pp. 302–329.

Fredrickson, B.L. (2003) The value of positive emotions. *American Scientist*, 91, 330–335.

Fredrickson, B. (2009) *Positivity*. New York: Crown Publishing Group.

George, B. (2004) *Authentic Leadership: rediscovering the secrets to creating lasting value*. Chichester: John Wiley & Sons.

Hallowell, E.M. (1999) The human moment at work. *Harvard Business Review*, 77(1), 58–64.

Hatfield, E., Cacioppo, J.T. and Rapson, R.L. (1994) *Emotional Contagion*. Cambridge: Cambridge University Press.

Hawkins, P. (2011) *Leadership Team Coaching: developing collective transformational leadership*. London: Kogan Page.

Hofstede, G., Neuijen, B., Ohayv, D. D. and Sanders, G. (1990) Measuring organizational cultures: a qualitative and quantitative study across twenty cases. *Administrative Science Quarterly*, 35(2), 286–316.

Kabat-Zinn, J. (1994) *Wherever You Go, There You Are*. London: Piatkus.

Kahn, W.A. (1990) Psychological conditions of personal engagement and disengagement at work. *Academy of Management Journal*, 33(4), 692–724.

Langer, E.J. and Rodin, J. (1976) The effects of choice and enhanced personal responsibility: a field experiment in an institutional setting. *Journal of Personality and Social Psychology*, 34, 191–198.

Miller, T. (1995) *How to Want What You Have: discovering the magic and grandeur of ordinary existence*. New York: Avon Books.

Nolen-Hoeksema, S. and Davis, C.G. (2004) Positive responses to loss. In: Snyder, C.R. and Lopez, S.J. (eds) *Handbook of Positive Psychology*. London: Oxford University Press, pp. 598–607.

Patterson, J. (2001) *Suzanne's Diary for Nicholas*. New York: Little, Brown.

Reivich, K. and Shatté, A. (2002) *The Resilience Factor: 7 essential skills for overcoming life's inevitable obstacles*. New York: Broadway Books.

Seligman, M.E.P. (1991) *Learned Optimism*. New York: Knopf.

Schwartz, T. and McCarthy, C. (2007) Manage your energy, not your time. *Harvard Business Review*, 85(10).

Stewart, I. and Joines, V. (1987) *TA Today*. Nottingham: Lifespace Publishing.

Tedeschi, R.G. and Calhoun, L.G. (2004) Posttraumatic growth: conceptual foundations and empirical evidence. *Psychological* Inquiry, 15(1), 1–18.

Wilson, T.D. (2002) *Strangers to Ourselves: discovering the adaptive unconscious*. Cambridge, MA: Harvard University Press.

Part 2

Leading others with skill

Chapter 4 **Getting my message across**

John Deffenbaugh

A number of years ago, Paul Newman starred in a well-known film called *Cool Hand Luke*. He played a prisoner who tried unsuccessfully on a number of occasions to escape, leading to an exchange with the prison warden, who observed 'What we've got here is failure to communicate'.

This pretty well sums up too many communication exchanges. Failure to communicate stems from many factors, such as lack of understanding of the other's position, lack of empathy, not appreciating the context, defensiveness – the list is endless, largely because communication is between people, and we're all different. The complaints process that patients go through often highlights that they simply want to hear an acknowledgement of the simplest, and most difficult, word in the English language – sorry.

This chapter is about communication as a nurse or midwife – getting your message across. The chapter addresses this challenge from three perspectives. First, knowing the audience – who you are communicating with. Second, the message that is being communicated. Third, a range of means for how your message can be put across.

Knowing your audience

There are two broad audiences that will be explored here – those who you serve and those you work with. Let's consider patients and service users first.

Communicating with patients
This area is a core skill for nurses and midwives. Yet to take communication skills for granted is to ignore the evidence of numerous reports on NHS

How to be a Nurse or Midwife Leader, First Edition.
Edited by David Ashton, Jamie Ripman and Philippa Williams.
© 2017 John Wiley & Sons, Ltd. Published 2017 by John Wiley & Sons, Ltd.

services. For example, the findings of Robert Francis (2010) into care at Mid Staffordshire NHS Foundation Trust:

> *'If there is one lesson to be learnt, I suggest that it is that people must always come before numbers. It is the individual experiences that lie behind statistics and benchmarks and action plans that really matter, and that is what must never be forgotten when policies are being made and implemented.'*

It is with this background in mind that this chapter begins with communication with patients. Patients and service users will be anxious, vulnerable, worried. They may well feel disempowered and angry – a wide range of emotions, often coming together in actions that may seem irrational but are perfectly reasonable given the circumstances. Nurses and midwives will have been trained in responding to these emotions but, in the heat of the moment, some of these core skills will not come to the fore – frankly, too, some nurses and midwives will be better communicators than others.

The families and carers of patients and service users may also feel this anxiety and disempowerment. In some cases they will magnify the patient's concerns, in other cases mollify them. Language may also be a barrier to communication, and may take away from the immediacy and effectiveness of response. This is where non-verbal communication comes to the fore – the touch, the expression, the tone of voice, even if the words are not understood.

Then there is the cultural sensitivity of this communication, both verbal and non-verbal. For some cultures there may be pressure to speak to family members instead of the patient, which adds a further complication to the process, though, of course, it may assist in providing the necessary care and attention.

Patient communication can, therefore, be one to one or with a family group. Either setting can be fraught with communication challenges, and in a family group there is a need to recognise and respond to the wider range of emotions that will be present. This may, of course, also be the case with the transition of emotions that a patient will go through over time as they understand their situation and respond to the information available to them.

Identify some colleagues with whom it feels possible for you to discuss those occasions when you know you have communicated effectively and how you knew this. Have that conversation and also discuss those times when you had a sense of your communication being a little clumsy, mistimed or less effective.

Some times we over- or undertransmit information and sometimes we don't receive it – consider what happened for you and what you think might have been the situation for the recipient.

Refer back to Chapter 2 where this topic is covered in depth.

As Elisabeth Kübler-Ross (1969) originally presented in her Five Stages of Grief, these emotions may begin with shock, then denial, moving onto blame and withdrawal before emerging as discovery and optimism for the future – this concept is covered further in Chapter 7. This is where clinical input comes to the fore – helping the patient and relatives along this transition curve (Fink *et al.*, 1971), allowing time to progress but providing prompts and challenges as appropriate. As Ron Heifetz and colleagues (2009) observed, 'What people resist is not change *per se*, but loss'. From a patient's perspective, this loss will come from their illness, their change in life circumstance, their feeling of disempowerment.

How a nurse or midwife leader engages with patients will obviously vary with the circumstances – each situation is unique. When commenting on these circumstances, one of our nurse leaders observed:

'When you are dealing with the very sick, the first piece of advice is to appear very clever. Get to know your speciality and discuss it in a way that sets you aside from the medics. Explain very clearly and relate it to the type of patient you are dealing with. A traveller will need very different information compared to a corporate lawyer and although not job specific, patients' and their relatives' expectations must be fully understood. Most importantly, information that is being shared should be true, relevant and at the level required and nurses should learn their specialities like the back of their hand to be fully appreciated by their patients.'

There is no uniform approach to communicating with a patient in these circumstances, since we are all individuals – patients and nurses – and the context will always vary. There are some approaches that we can consider, however, to obtain guidance on how best to get the message across. Ezekiel and Linda Emanuel (1992) looked at four models of clinician–patient relationship.

- *Paternalistic* – clinician has a parental role, deciding which treatment is best.
- *Informative* – clinician tells patients about treatment options and relevant medical information.
- *Interpretative* – clinician helps patients explore their values.
- *Deliberative* – clinician helps patients explore health-related values.

The approach taken by a nurse has a direct impact on outcome. Over recent decades there has been a shift to the informative approach, especially as patients can now find information about their condition on the internet, which repositions patients as partners in the treatment process. This can be combined with the deliberative approach, which guides patients in a caring manner but does not limit their independence.

Information should never be allowed to remain hidden, as a nurse leader observed.

> 'This requires intuition and then some direct and open questioning. I think that many nurses try to avoid difficult communication scenarios with either their patients or relatives and this tends to build barriers. Nurses of all grades should look for dissatisfied patients and ask them how they can help to improve their experience. Without asking, some people will never disclose, but if they feel you are concerned about them because you have asked, then the following conversations will be fluid and much easier than they would have been if ignored. This often gives nurses the ability to rectify small issues such as diet requirements, but also can escalate when patients are becoming more unwell. This approach can diffuse a rumbling feud in an instant. If patients and relatives trust you as a nurse, then their entire hospital stay will inevitably be problem free. Minor complaints must be addressed prior to the complaint itself and it takes "forward planning communication" to achieve this. There is no science behind a health care professional saying something like, "Hi Mr Smith, you don't seem as happy today, is there anything wrong?". All too often when nurses suspect something is wrong or someone is dissatisfied, the patient or relative is temporarily blanked until a distraction replaces their dissatisfaction.'

After the initial Francis Inquiry (2010) into Mid Staffordshire NHS Foundation Trust, the NHS England Chief Nursing Officer Jane Cummings used the framework of the 6Cs to focus the profession on the 'basics' for excellence in nursing and midwifery (Cummings and Bennett, 2012). One of the 6Cs of nursing is Compassion: 'how care is given through relationships based on empathy, respect and dignity'. This frames the communication process, so that patients feel the compassion for their condition from the nurse or midwife – in addition to the nurse feeling the need to demonstrate that they are 'clever'. One of our nurse leaders reflected on their early career.

> 'Communication as a new, and occasionally scared, qualified nurse or midwife is crucial in the lines of development, rapport building with staff and, of course, patient engagement and safety. I think the rules are loosely edged as a lot of good communication comes down to character.'

This balanced relationship with patients is therefore underpinned by effective conversation. The same is true with colleagues – to change behaviour of patients, it is first necessary to change behaviour of clinicians.

Communicating with colleagues

Nurse and midwife leaders have a pivotal role in engaging staff to be partners in the patient care process. By their communication – verbal and non-verbal – they set the scene for how effective the team is; they put in place the culture of care, namely 'how we do things around here'. As with patient interaction, it is essential to get into the shoes of staff, to see it from their perspective – which indeed was the position they used to be in before they became a nurse leader.

Nurse and midwife leaders will communicate in a range of settings: one to one, small group and larger presentations. The approach taken for each setting will vary, of course, but there are some common and inter-related themes.

First is the *authenticity* with which a nurse or midwife leader communicates. Rob Goffee and Gareth Jones (2005) have written extensively about authenticity; other contributors to this book will also cover authenticity and it is something worthy of a little repetition. Goffee and Jones define authenticity as 'a quality that others must attribute to you'. They continue, 'The ability to strike the balance between expressing their personalities and managing those of the people they aspire to lead is what distinguishes great leaders from other executives'.

There are three components to authenticity. First is knowing yourself. You need to be comfortable in your own skin – who you are, where you came from, your comfort zones and preparedness to receive honest feedback. As a nurse or midwife leader, the challenge for you will be to get outside these comfort zones, to see things differently and build mental agility to embrace change.

Second is getting to know your staff. There is a fine line here between what to divulge to staff and what you want divulged from them. Part of understanding this will be insight into the context in which you are operating – the ward, department, service. Your behaviours and actions can remove barriers between yourself and others, allowing you to empathise compassionately with your colleagues, letting others know what is unique and authentic about them. The extent of this communication – disclosure, questioning, listening – will depend on who you are engaging with and the circumstances you are in. Suffice to say, appropriate disclosure is somewhere in the large space between, at worst, putting up a 'brick wall' and, at the opposite extreme, becoming too familiar.

Finally, there is making the connection to the organisational context. At this stage you will be getting the right distance between you and colleagues, sharpening your social antennae to determine how this is received, and showing by your behaviour that you honour deeply held values and social mores. As one of our nurse leaders commented about the means used for authenticity:

> '*Impromptu encounters are as important as the planned ones for getting the message across to staff – informal ones are as important as formal.*'

However, sometimes you may be setting out to change the behaviours of others, if they are counter-cultural to the aims of the organisation or the team. For this you'll need to develop the resilience that we explored in the last chapter.

Rather than replicating that, we cross-refer you to the insight of Karen Reivich and Andrew Shatté (2003) who observed that 'resilience is not only about overcoming, it is also about the ability to enhance the positive aspects of our lives'. You will therefore bring all aspects of your life into your work. Some leaders are better at compartmentalisation than others, but there will of necessity be some overlap. Home and work can too readily become one, whether for you as a nurse leader or for the staff you lead.

These resilience factors link with the third theme that underpins your communication with staff, which is the *values* that you hold and exhibit as a leader. The NHS Constitution provides the framework for the values that NHS staff should hold. In exhibiting these, you will have your own set of values – the direction in which your personal compass points (see exercises in Chapter 3).

> Take some time to read (or re-read) at least the opening section of the NHS Constitution. It is a powerful message about values and the commitment the NHS makes to the people who have need of its services and the staff who work in it.

Values-based leadership is about motivating employees by connecting organisational goals to employees' personal values. As Harry Kraemer (2011) observed, some of the traits of values-based leaders are self-reflection, balance, self-confidence and humility. These link back to the authenticity you exhibit and the resilience you hold.

The alignment of values must be both down and across the organisation. As a values-based leader, you will be communicating organisational values that tell colleagues how to behave in order to meet the needs of the patients you serve and the organisation in which you work. These values could be based around the 6Cs of nursing and midwifery: Care, Compassion, Competence, Communication, Courage, Commitment.

You may find that there is a disconnect between these values and the circumstances in which you are operating. For instance, pressure on staffing levels or procedures you are asked to follow may conflict with your view of how you provide services in the best interest of your patients. In cases such as these, your professional judgement comes into play, as well as your skills in managing upwards. This is where the value of feedback comes to the fore, as one of our nurse leaders observed.

> '*As a fairly reflective individual, I underestimated the impact this would have – to see yourself as others see you can be uncomfortable but also powerful. It is important to have insight in to what staff/patients want from you as an individual or as part of a service and the value they place on that.*'

You will need to talk about these values in a way that connects with the personal values of nurse and midwife colleagues, so that they come to identify strongly with both the organisation and its objectives, not just the department or ward in which you work. As a middle leader in the organisation, you hold the values in your hands. You will therefore need to focus on core values – the enduring guiding principles that capture the organisation's strengths and character. Because the core values represent the soul of the organisation, they are likely to remain steadfast in the face of changing market trends and fads.

Gerry Johnson and Kevan Scholes (1998) developed the Culture Web as an effective way of capturing these values, as illustrated in Figure 4.1. The six

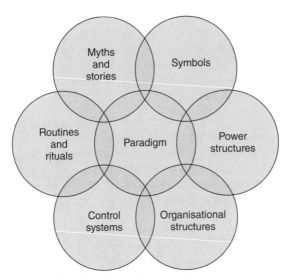

Figure 4.1 The Culture Web. Source: Johnson, G. and Scholes, K. (1998) *Exploring Corporate Strategy*. Harlow: Prentice Hall. Reproduced with permission of Pearson Education Ltd.

elements of the Culture Web illustrate both the 'soft' (symbols, myths and stories, routines and rituals) and the 'hard' (control systems, organisational structures, power structures) elements that make up the cultural paradigm – 'the way we do things around here'.

The way in which you, as nurse leader, act and behave will set the scene for effective communication. In your own communication, you will tell certain stories that resonate, follow routines and rituals, and use symbols to reinforce your message. Equally, you will put in place reporting lines and control measures that either enhance or limit communication.

This Culture Web tool can be used at departmental level, not just organisationally, though it will, of course, be expected to align in many respects. It can also be used to change culture, since you may find that what is in place is not suitable to meet the needs of patients.

In order for staff to believe in the sincerity and depth of your and the organisation's values, you must lead by example and communicate the values on an ongoing basis to the staff who work for you and to those who work alongside your team. You can therefore get your message across not just by conversation but by the wider range of 'soft' and 'hard' levers at your disposal.

Finally, there is your style of *influencing* as a means of communication. One of our nurse leaders commented:

> 'The value of "making every conversation count" has stuck with me. I don't see any encounter as too "small". For example, using opportunities in various forums to participate, influence or motivate others, such as bed meetings (isolation priorities), new build meetings (trying new materials), non-exec and patient governors meetings (hearing concerns, providing updates/assurance).'

In Chapter 6 we explore the styles and skills of influencing in depth, and we'll return to this aspect of getting your message across then.

In all our communications, it is vitally important to know your audience – what will cause them to be influenced effectively by you? Part of the answer to this question lies in the message that you as a leader are seeking to communicate. We now address this aspect of communicating.

Framing the message

To paraphrase St Paul in his first epistle to the Corinthians, 'nobody follows an uncertain trumpet'. The impact model discussed in Chapter 2 provides a framework for the effective communication of a message. People are not machines so conversation is vital, in whatever context. Narrative leadership is the art of telling a coherent and convincing story – one that acknowledges where an organisation has come from, recognises the realities of the present situation, and offers a worthwhile future. An authentic leader will bring something of themselves into this story, making a connection with the people who hear the story.

In considering the message that a nurse or midwife leader will convey, let's consider first your leadership style – then, how your story is constructed.

Leadership style

There is a range of ways to describe leadership style, and one of the more evidence-based approaches draws on the work of Daniel Goleman (2000), who summarises six leadership styles as follows.

- *Affiliative* – 'Let's do what's best for everyone'
- *Coaching* – 'How can I help you do it better?'
- *Directive* – 'Do what I tell you'
- *Pacesetting* – 'Do what I do'
- *Participative* – 'Let's decide what to do together'
- *Visionary* – 'Do what will help us reach our goals'

The aim should be that nurse leaders exhibit a range of leadership styles, but mainly use those that encourage a positive organisation climate. However, diagnostic work with NHS leaders (Santry, 2012) has shown that they tend towards a limited range of styles, and lean towards pacesetting style, which has a negative impact on climate. This stems largely from the prevailing culture in the NHS, which is target driven, with the urgent being acted on over the important, and leaders feeling like they are on a treadmill of activity and action. When they pause and get off – because they have not previously taken the time to set a vision, engage and coach staff – nurse and midwife leaders can too readily default to the directive leadership style, which also has a negative impact on organisation climate. The result is that short-term targets are met but staff are not engaged, so performance lacks sustainability.

One of our nurse leaders commented on his leadership and communication style.

> 'The more senior you become in nursing, the more difficult the questions become, coupled with delivery issues due to the widening scope of your job. You will be busier than ever and need to section time out for good communication with patients during your busy schedule. Zoning in on each patient you are responsible for does not take much time, but there must be adequate engagement. Patients and relatives will expect all healthcare professionals to be more direct than themselves in most situations, and this must be fully understood.'

The lessons are clear. Nurse leaders should develop a range of styles, including pacesetting and directive where appropriate, but mainly use ones that set the vision for staff, embrace them in achieving the goals, and coach them in quality service provision. For this, it is essential to have a leadership narrative.

Leadership narrative

Stories and narratives are important because they are the primary way we make sense of our experience, creating (and recreating) our sense of self – who we are and what we stand for. They are a vital means of building relationships, bringing together (and dividing) groups and communities. Stories are a powerful force in the world, shaping, constraining and freeing our sense of what is desirable and possible. Reflecting back on our own childhood, we often recall the stories we were read at bedtime, and the impact they had.

In organisational life, and for nurse and midwife leaders, stories can be laden with implicit value-judgements. The culture of an organisation and the person-ality of the leader are both reflected in, and shaped by, the stories that are told.

A very effective tool through which a story can be framed is the structure of a public narrative, which has been developed by Marshal Ganz (2009). This model of public narrative is illustrated in Figure 4.2.

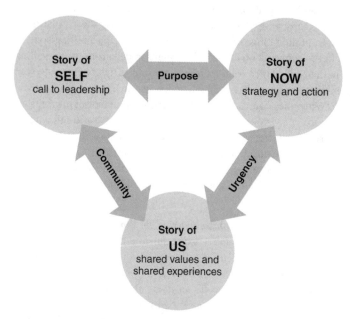

Figure 4.2 Model of public narrative. Source: Reproduced with permission of Marshall Ganz.

A public narrative has three elements.

- *Story of self* – a story about why you are called to leadership that enables others to understand you and the values that you hold.
- *Story of us* – a story about the values and aspirations of your community and the experiences, good or bad, that demonstrate them.
- *Story of now* – a story about the urgent challenge that you hope to inspire others to take action on.

This framework plays well to nurse and midwife leaders, who passionately talk about their call to nursing. This gives point to the call to leadership, and links with purpose in calling staff in their nurse community to action with a sense of urgency. Marshall Ganz in this context refers to leadership as 'taking responsibility for enabling others to achieve shared purpose in the face of uncertainty'.

A narrative focuses on winning the heart – this is why young children so love stories, and why adults become very adept at telling stories. However, some of these story-telling skills are lost, or misplaced, when it comes to the workplace. Maybe they're seen as less relevant, maybe there is not the time, or probably the time is not created. Maybe also there is a need for confidence building about how to tell stories to adults.

Stories therefore have something to offer in motivating others to join us in action. This can be understood by considering the different ways in which we understand the world around us, the challenges we face and the action we might take. Psychologists tell us that we are capable of understanding the world in two distinct ways – the 'head' mode and the 'heart' mode; this links again to the skill of influencing which we'll explore in Chapter 6.

The *head* mode helps us with strategy and analysis. It helps us to answer 'how' questions. How should we deliver patient care or plan the shift? Leadership obviously requires these skills but we often act as if this is the only way of understanding the world around us. When we are trying to seek support, we tend to believe that if only we could find the right argument or piece of evidence, surely others would come around to our way of thinking.

One of the reasons why this often fails is because it misses out the second way in which we look at the world – the *heart* mode. This mode helps us to understand the world in a completely different way – in terms of whether things are good or bad for us, hopeful or depressing, attractive or repulsive. The heart mode helps us to answer the 'why' questions. Why should I care about how my colleague feels when I give feedback? Winning over the heart is the domain of story telling rather than strategy and analysis.

Effective leadership requires both these modes, the head and the heart, in order to move the *hands* – which is to move others to action. The heart mode helps us to understand what we value – but how does this help us to move people to action? The answer lies in understanding the link between values, emotion and action that is central to public narrative. Values inspire action through emotion. Our emotions provide information to the mind about what it is that we value.

People who are unable to feel emotion are also unable to make choices. This is especially important in story telling through public narrative because ultimately you will be asking people to make a choice to join you in action. Unless you can provide them with the emotional information they need, they are unlikely to do so.

Nurse and midwife leaders will find themselves in the positon of engaging staff, colleagues, patients and relatives on a daily basis. Using appropriate leadership styles, you will want to call on the skills of story telling and the form of public narrative when the circumstances are right. You will also need to be aware of what enables effective public narrative, and what inhibits it. Therefore, emotions that are 'action motivators' need to come to the fore to counter emotions that are 'action inhibitors', which include:

- *turning apathy to anger* – if the people you are hoping to move to action are feeling apathetic, you need to give them the experience of feeling outrage to provide the emotional information they need to enable them to make the choice to join you
- *turning isolation to solidarity* – if the people you are hoping to move to action are feeling isolated, you need to give them the experience of feeling their connectedness with others to enable them to make the choice to join you.

When you are developing your public narrative, you are seeking to promote those emotions that motivate others in order to help overcome the emotions that most often inhibit us from taking action. One of our nurse leaders contributed his observations about engaging with patients.

'*A lot of patients come into hospital feeling very nervous and anxious. Laughter, used in the correct way, is essential in building solid communication lines between patients and nurses. Most patients want a light-hearted approach most of the time and if this is deployed, the rewards are plentiful. Patients tend to complain more about nurses not engaging with them than anything else. You will hear them say, "that night nurse was a right misery last night" or "she was very good but she didn't really talk to me". These will be informal complaints or snippets from shifts in the past. If you engage with your patients directly, with a smile and occasionally with some laughter, when you are absent patients will simply ask every member of staff on the ward when you are next on shift.'*

Stories in a public narrative have a structure, similar to the stories we all recall from our childhood.

- *Character* – or set of characters who are central to the story.
- *Plot* – the guts of the story that comprises the challenge, the choice and the outcome.
- *Moral* – the lessons from the choice we make to face the challenge and achieve the desired outcome.

With a good story you lean in a bit, because you are curious. A tear might come to the eye, the hairs bristle at the back of the neck. You realise you care, because with stories that connect with us emotionally we are able to experience the courage, fear, hope of the protagonist.

Give it a go! There is no single way to frame or present a public narrative. Give yourself some time to work with the Marshal Ganz structure and tailor it to your own context – who you are, who you're seeking to influence, what it is that you are asking them to do. You might want to have a core message that is conveyed in a number of ways, and tailored to the specific circumstance. For instance, at the start of a meeting or hand-over, you may draw on a set of core themes that you keep reinforcing, with other points to address specifics of that moment. In this way, you have the best of both worlds – you reinforce the values you wish to see in staff, and communicate the message of the moment. The 6Cs that we referred to earlier are a good example of core nursing messages that can be built into your public narrative.

Let's now move onto the range of circumstances in which the message can be communicated.

Context for communicating the message

As a nurse or midwife leader, there will be many circumstances where you have to get your message across. While there are some best practice principles that are relevant to all circumstances, it is vitally important to tailor the message to the audience in front of you. We therefore discuss here how to tailor your message to your audience in a number of different situations. First, however, let's explore some common best practice communication themes.

Best practice communication tips

It is always helpful to have a number of core best practice points you can draw on as you communicate in any circumstance. Linking back to some of the areas we focused on in Chapter 2, these include the following.

- *Posture* – hold yourself erect and if sitting don't slump in a chair
- *Eye contact* – with the people you are communicating to, not the ceiling
- *Breathing* – steady, in-out, pausing to catch breath
- *Voice* – range of pitch, rather than monotone
- *Emphasis of words* – to make key messages stand out
- *Pace/pause* – using silence as a powerful tool
- *Mindfulness* – being aware of self and the world around you

Some of these skills will need to be practised, and confidence will come with time. You may already feel more confident in some of these areas than others. The point is that these best practice tips are universal in the interactions you have with others, whether in a work setting, at home or with friends. However, in your role as a nurse or midwife leader, let's explore some of the settings in which you will be communicating your message to see how you might tailor it further to the specific context.

Team meeting

Earlier in this chapter we discussed approaches to communicating with colleagues. A common means for this communication is the team meeting. These can range from formal to informal, and a recent variant is the 'team huddle'.

Team meetings act as a means of reinforcing key messages, aspects of culture that are important, and what is necessary to meet the needs of patients. Team meetings are often given less attention than they deserve. They reinforce the concept of 'the team' and, as presented by Jon Katzenbach and Douglas Smith (1993), teams offer a number of benefits. They:

- bring together complementary skills and experiences that exceed those of any individual, enabling a better response to multifaceted challenges
- establish communications that support real-time problem solving and initiative, jointly developing clear goals and approaches
- can adjust their approach to new information and challenges with greater speed, accuracy and effectiveness
- provide a unique social dimension that enhances the economic and administrative aspects of work, overcoming the barriers that stand in the way of collective performance.

West *et al.* (2014) provide insight into 'real team' criteria, one of which is that real teams meet regularly to review performance and take corrective action, based on having clear objectives and working closely to achieve these objectives.

Team meetings therefore become the means of leveraging enhanced team performance, and a means for a nurse or midwife leader to get their message across and convey their values.

These meetings are also another means of engaging staff. It is the 'voices from below' who often have insight into patient issues and how to solve them. Team meetings then become a vehicle for meeting the criteria of effective employee engagement explored by David MacLeod and Nita Clark (2009):

- a strategic narrative that links staff to the organisation
- engaging managers who communicate this narrative
- enabling the employee voice
- building organisation integrity in the eyes of stakeholders.

There are a number of ways in which team meetings can be improved, leading to both more effective team working and performance outcomes. Best practice includes:

- setting a regular time and sticking to it
- holding meetings in an environment conducive to open discussion
- switching off phones/tablets so that staff can 'be there'
- having a clear agenda that can be covered during the meeting
- prioritising agenda items so that the important does not get swamped by the urgent
- providing a balanced chair role that both enables discussion and moves things forward
- maximising the listening time for the views of staff, not projecting own views or solutions
- building responsibility for ownership by staff of the problems and solutions
- keeping the patient in the forefront of discussion
- recording actions and timeframes
- revisiting what has been agreed to ensure implementation.

Take some time to consider the meetings you attend or possibly lead. How well do they fit with best practice? What steps will you take to make sure that they do?

Not all staff will be able to be present for team meetings and, indeed, with technology and virtual working nowadays, the days of physical presence may be numbered. Certainly, for community-based teams that may be spread over a wide geographic area, video or telephone conferencing may be the standard format for meetings. In this case, there are a number of further best practice tips for effectiveness.

- Ensure you are in a quiet environment, as background noises are a real distraction.
- Firm chairing that invites participants to contribute and ensures balanced participation.
- Not talking over colleagues and practising brevity.
- Not getting distracted by other things in your setting.

Reflecting on meetings and staff engagement, one of our nurse leaders observed:

> 'Repeating the message is often necessary. Start on the premise that everyone has something valuable to contribute and there is good in everyone. Be enthusiastic. Nurture positive working relationships. Always stay in "adult" mode so that you are communicating with people who are "adults".Show care for staff – they are more likely to listen. See staff as people who have had their own "journeys", and a weekend to ask about, for example.'

Effective teams and team meetings go hand in hand. It is challenging to build teamwork without some form of team interaction. It should, of course, take place on a day-to-day level, and not wait for the formal meeting, since patients expect nurses to work as an integrated team, to communicate, hand over, and share patient experience. One of the things that really exasperates patients is to have to continually repeat their story – 'don't they speak to each other?' is too often the view of patients when referring to nurses and other staff.

Chairing a meeting

The chair's role is integral to effective team meetings, and one of the key ingredients of chairing is active listening.

- Give people your full attention – not becoming distracted or getting called away.
- Make it clear that you are listening – demonstrate body language that communicates this.
- Be ready to paraphrase or 'play back' – to 'join the dots' in discussion to see the bigger picture.
- If you do not understand, ask – seek clarity of the views.
- Acknowledge the other person's feelings – there may be passion that needs to be recognised and channelled.
- Encourage the other person if they appear uncertain – provide space for everyone to contribute.

- Do not respond until the other person has finished – but, equally, move things on if they get ground into the sand.
- Beware of passing judgement too quickly – keep an open mind.

Effective chairing is about enabling others to contribute, and through this allowing staff to both solve problems and take ownership, rather than imposing your views. However, it is also important for the chair to summarise the points made, and move to a decision if necessary.

Chairing is more about enquiring than advocating. It is about exploring others' points of views and the reasons behind them, and focusing on the topic at hand rather than getting distracted. It may be that there is some advocacy around the context, or the urgency of the situation that requires command and control, but this is probably the exception rather than the rule. The balance of advocacy and inquiry is to show curiosity, to make reasoning explicit, to ask others about assumptions, without being critical or accusing. This is the chair's skilful role to generate ideas through the effectiveness of team work.

Chairing a meeting is therefore about both efficiency and effectiveness. Efficiency comes from setting an agenda that can be covered in the time available, enabling all to contribute as appropriate, keeping to time, summing up and moving things along. You therefore want to tick the box that says the meeting proceeded according to plan (or close to it).

Many leaders regard efficiency as the measure of success for a meeting. Certainly, if a meeting runs over, has an agenda that is too onerous or lacks firm chairing, then participants will go away less than satisfied. But meetings also need to be effective. This means that there needs to be some flexibility in discussing issues that reflect their importance, all views are aired, the chair does not dominate discussion, conclusions are reached, and action is agreed. Meetings are valuable commodities, and it is worth reflecting on the advice of Peter Drucker (1966): 'One either meets or one works. One cannot do both at the same time'.

Before chairing your next meeting, read through this section of the chapter again and make some specific notes about what you will do to chair the meeting well. Take a bit more time to prepare and, after the meeting, reflect on any differences this makes to the outcome of the meeting and how you are perceived.

Presentation

There will be occasions when as a nurse or midwife leader you will be asked to give a presentation – indeed, you may want to use a presentation format to get your point across.

It is important to recognise at the outset that presentation does not mean PowerPoint. The spoken word in itself is very powerful, and PowerPoint is but one means of enhancing the words you will utter. At their worst, PowerPoint presentations distract from the message conveyed, and reduce impact. At their best, they can provide a memorable event.

There are three ingredients to successful presentation – knowing your audience, knowing your material, conveying the message.

First, know your *audience*. You may be familiar with who you are presenting to, but do you know their expectations for the presentation? What are they looking for? Who has influence? What is the outcome you want, the audience wants? Audiences are generally not out to trip you up, and are really willing you to succeed – to use the presentation to help move their agenda forward. If you have not done your homework on what they are looking for, however, you may trip yourself up.

Secondly, know your *material*. You are giving the presentation because you are perceived to know something that would be useful to the audience. If this is not the case, consider someone else giving the presentation with you in support. You need to know your material, as this will enable discussion and questions to flow naturally, and for you to demonstrate your knowledge and insight. Have notes at hand, but don't be a slave to them.

Finally, how you choose to convey your *message* will go a considerable way towards a successful outcome. The 'tyranny of PowerPoint' is as much on you as it is the audience – material that is too dense to read, badly presented, and way too many slides. Yes, a 'picture tells a thousand words' so you don't need a thousand pictures. Less can be more in these circumstances, so the spoken word should come to the fore, with slides to illustrate and act as an *aide-mémoire* for the discussion. This approach also enables flexibility of presentation and an ability to tailor to the audience.

Here are some best practice tips on preparing, designing and delivering an effective presentation.

Preparation
- Clarity on the objective for the presentation – what you want achieve
- Insight into your audience and their expectations
- Deep understanding of your content
- Build your confidence with thorough preparation

Design
- Simplification of your message – what are the key points you wish to convey?
- Clear, logical structure with signposts – tell a story

- Effective choice of illustration, visual or stories
- Plan your logical points – follow the 'elevator test' of getting across your message in a short period

Delivery
- Plan a confident start
- Use visuals to shift attention to give yourself space
- Connect with the audience through eye contact and body language
- Keep to message

One straightforward way to frame and deliver your presentation is to think of yourself in the audience. What would you want to hear? What would impress you? What does not impress you? All too often, we lose this connection with ourselves and view a presentation in the abstract. We are one of them, so get into the shoes of the audience.

As with the best practice tips, there are certainly some things to avoid.

- Standing in front of the screen
- Jingling coins in your pocket
- Mumbling and speaking too softly
- Being unnecessarily flippant
- Speaking to the ceiling, or one person
- Telling inappropriate jokes
- Not valuing your audience

> As with most things in life, practice makes perfect. Rehearse your next presentation in front of the mirror to see yourself in action. In addition, before your next presentation, test it out with a work colleague, friend, partner or son/daughter. Choose someone who will be your most effective critical friend and try out your presentation as if you were giving it to your real audience.

Board paper and meeting
Communicating by board paper, or other type of discussion paper, is a particular challenge. Nurse and midwife leaders may not be particularly trained in the art of writing, and it is indeed an art. Key to preparing a good paper is the outline – putting in place the logical structure, with signposts, that allows the reader to follow the flow of discussion to the logical conclusion that you are seeking to lead them towards.

When considering getting your message across in this setting, one of our nurse leaders reflected:

> '*It is important to be aware of organisational as well as individual priorities, what are the "levers" – is the chief executive motivated by achieving our*

(very tight) financial targets (among other things?). For different individuals and organisations this may differ. When asked, "What do we need to achieve this?", be prepared, share what the barriers are, offer solutions if you can, take the opportunity to drive change. We were able to secure funding for an extra member of staff and an IC database last year.'

There are a few best practice approaches that nurse and midwife leaders can follow when preparing a paper for a board presentation. First is the need to turn data into information. The NHS is not short of data, but this is all too seldom turned into information, and then knowledge, intelligence and insight as illustrated in Figure 4.3.

If you are presenting statistics, then interpret these. Do not just put a set of figures in a report, but rather tell the reader what this says. With multiple sets of tables and data, then 'join the dots' to provide an overview of what you take from the data. This takes balcony thinking, and if you do not carry this out, then the board will lack insight and might take the wrong tack in their questioning.

A second best practice tip for board papers is brevity. Sadly, many board papers are measured by what can be called the 'thud factor', namely the sound they make when dropped from a height and hit the floor.

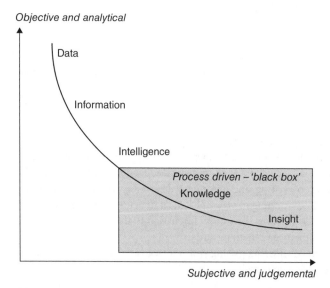

Figure 4.3 Turning data into information. Source: Reproduced with permission of Frontline.

Aim for a low thud factor. Board papers and other discussion papers are often way too long. It was the French mathematician and scientist, Blaise Pascal, who observed, 'I have made this letter longer than usual because I lack the time to make it short'. (This quote has also been attributed to many others!)

So make the time for good thinking and planning before you write. Prepare an outline, a storyboard, of what you want to say. This allows you to self-critique, and to keep to the plot. If you do not do this, then a paper grows arms and legs and you truly lose the plot.

A structure can help, and one with four elements keeps the board paper short.

- *Issue* – what is this about?
- *Facts* – give clarity to the issue
- *Reasoning* – the points you then need to make about the issue and facts
- *Recommendations* – what you are asking for

This structure can fit on one page, and both Winston Churchill and Ronald Reagan demanded that papers put in front of them contained this information on one page. While you need to think harder, it saves rewriting *War and Peace*, and the paper will engage board members who do not really want to read a tome.

Finally, a third best practice tip is to find out about your audience. This was touched on earlier in this chapter, and the particular issue with board presentations is that the non-executives on the board perform what is called the 'challenge function', namely they bring their independent judgement and critical detachment to challenge what is put before them for consideration, discussion and decision making. Hence, you will need to prepare not just the paper but also your knowledge of the interests of the board and its members. What has been discussed before? Where do they stand on the issue? What are their expectations?

You will then need to be on your toes for the presentation itself. As discussed earlier, do not overcomplicate the presentation, and therefore waste the limited time available to you. Practise with a colleague, and make sure you set out the structure of the presentation at the start, then present the content, followed by the summing up with your key messages. Consider using the public narrative approach presented earlier to make a connection with board members. When questions follow, be prepared. If you do not know, say so and follow up with the answer after the meeting. Board members will not usually set out to trip you up but if you are not prepared, you may trip yourself up. Carry out your own challenge function in advance, which will make the board's challenge more effective, leading to a beneficial outcome.

Conclusion

There are no secrets to getting your message across. Nurse and midwife leaders will do this in many settings outside work – at home, in groups and social circles, and through daily activities such as shopping. Communication is an art, not a science, though, as presented in this chapter, there are a number of methods and approaches that you can follow which will help you in your artistry. Being self-aware enables you to be a better communicator, and elsewhere in this book you will learn about the impact you have on others, how to build your resilience, and how to read the context in which you are communicating. Be open to feedback on how your message is received, and avoid getting into the situation where you are told that 'What we have here is a failure to communicate'.

References

Cummings, J. and Bennett, V. (2012) *Compassion in Practice: nursing, midwifery and care staff – our strategy*. Leeds: NHS England.

Drucker, P. (1966) *The Effective Executive*. New York: HarperCollins.

Emanuel, E.J. and Emanuel, L.L. (1992) Four models of the physician–patient relationship. *Journal of the American Medical Association*, V267(16), 2221–2226.

Fink, L.S., Beak, J. and Taddeo, K. (1971) Organisational crisis and change. *Journal of Applied Behavioural Science*, 7(1), 15–37.

Francis, R. (2010) *Independent Inquiry into Care Provided by Mid Staffordshire NHS Foundation Trust: January 2005–March 2009*. London: Stationery Office.

Ganz, M. (2009) Why stories matter – the art and craft of social change. *Sojourners*, March, 18–19.

Goffee, R. and Jones, G. (2005) Managing authenticity: the paradox of great leadership. *Harvard Business Review*, 83(12), 86–94.

Goleman, D. (2000) Leadership that gets results. *Harvard Business Review*, 78(2), 78–79.

Heifetz, R., Grashow, G. and Linsky, M. (2009) *The Practice of Adaptive Leadership: tools and tactics for changing your organization and the world*. Boston, MA: Harvard Business School Publishing.

Johnson, G. and Scholes, K. (1998) *Exploring Corporate Strategy*. Harlow: Prentice Hall.

Katzenback, J. and Smith, D. (1993) *The Wisdom of Teams: creating the high performance organisation*. New York: HarperCollins.

Kraemer, H. (2011) *From Values to Action: the four principles of values-based leadership*. San Francisco, CA: Jossey-Bass.

Kübler-Ross, E. (1969) *On Death and Dying*. New York: Scribner.

MacLeod, D. and Clarke, N. (2009) *Engaging for Success: enhancing performance through employee engagement*. London: Department for Business, Innovation and Skills.

Reivich, K. and Shatté, A. (2003) *The Resilience Factor: 7 keys to finding your inner strength and overcoming life's hurdles.* New York: Broadway Books.

Santry, C. (2012) Most senior leaders failing to create 'strong work climates. *Health Service Journal*, 122(6289), 9.

West, M.A., Lyubovnikova, J., Eckert, R. and Denis, J-L. (2014) Collective leadership for cultures of high quality health care. *Journal of Organizational Effectiveness: People and Performance*, v1(3), 240–260.

Chapter 5 **Getting the best out of others**

Alex Pett

With one junior nurse and a healthcare assistant, Rachel was working a shift on an elderly care ward with 26 patients, some of whom were at the end of life stage and needed a lot of support. There were clearly too few staff for the needs of the patients, but the whole hospital was struggling with staffing and the high demand for beds in winter. They were only just managing to stay on top of the requirements of the patients. Then a senior colleague arrived at the ward and said Rachel needed to take another patient. Rachel paused and then said no, she would not take the patient as the ward was already at maximum demand and it would not be safe to take another patient. The colleague said that if she did not take the patient, she would escalate this to more senior colleagues. Rachel explained politely but still refused.

Within 10 minutes Rachel received a phone call from a leadership team member who said that she must take this patient. Rachel then described the moment when she was about to agree to this demand, and just then some of her learning from the leadership programme came to mind. During the small group work, she had come to realise how she had a fundamental need for people to approve of her, to appreciate her hard work and to see her as kind and considerate. She also recognised that this led to her saying 'yes' to people too often, which meant she had a tendency to take on too much work and this could put her at risk. In that moment she knew she needed to say 'no'.

Rachel replied:

> 'I understand why you are asking me to take the patient but my answer is no. I am not going to discuss it on the phone because I have patients who need support right now. I am saying no because it will be unsafe for the patient and increase risk for those already in our care on this ward. If you want to discuss it you can come down to the ward and talk here.'

How to be a Nurse or Midwife Leader, First Edition.
Edited by David Ashton, Jamie Ripman and Philippa Williams.
© 2017 John Wiley & Sons, Ltd. Published 2017 by John Wiley & Sons, Ltd.

Having put the phone down. Rachel took a deep breath, smiled at her own self-assertion and went back to her patients.

The senior manager she spoke with on the phone was on the ward within 10 minutes along with two other senior managers. But Rachel was busy caring for patients, some who needed careful attention given their state of discomfort and pain, so she did not break away to talk with the senior colleagues. After around 20 minutes of waiting, the senior managers left the ward. At the end of the shift, the senior manager who had called Rachel called again, but this time to apologise for the inappropriate pressure they had put her under, and to say that Rachel had done the right thing.

Rachel's learning on the programme has been one of deeper self-awareness, understanding how she was at times meeting her own emotional needs rather than doing what was right for the situation. In this moment, this learning became an act of leadership in service of the patients under her care. But as much as this was an important breakthrough for Rachel, the problem here is that individual acts of leadership are not enough to change the performance of the health service. When the working environment is one of pressure, conflict, disagreement, constant change and at times chaos, significant and sustainable improvement in the quality and compassion of patient care requires many things, one of which is greater collective leadership.

This chapter is about how you develop a team of 'Rachels' – teams and groups of colleagues who are more likely to act effectively and with collective power. To explore this theme, we'll cover the need to know yourself as a leader, to be aware of those you work with, how to set a team up for success, and how humility is central to getting the best out of others.

- Introduction: being authentic
- Who we are and how we are
- Perception versus reality
- Working with others
- Setting up teams to perform well
- The power of humility

Introduction: being authentic

The late Aiden Halligan, former Deputy Chief Medical Officer for England, spoke regularly on one of the NHS Leadership Academy's programmes. On one of these occasions, I heard him use the phrase 'be the best of you on the worst of days'. This struck me as a deeply helpful way of thinking about the responsibility of a leader, how you can make the best contribution in your role, whatever the circumstances. I think this offers a great framework for leadership development, to participate in development work so we can be at our best in tough circumstances.

> This then raises all sorts of questions, including 'what is "you" at your best? '. How do you tend to behave when you are not at your best? When does this typically happen and do you know why? How are you helping others be at their best even in tough circumstances?
>
> You could consider these questions on your own, or even better with a group of colleagues.

The role of the leader is not simply to maintain the status quo but to bring about positive change through others, in a way that will improve the quality of care. I think a leader should be able to answer these questions and be seeking to be the best 'them' through development, reflection and feedback. A part of development is to know clearly what behaviours and ways of working are you 'at your best', and either what is you at your 'worst' or simply your behaviours that are unhelpful for leading.

Participants on programmes who are earlier in their career often express an expectation that they need to be like other leaders. However, I think at the heart of leadership is the need to be authentic – to see how your own personality and values create a style of leadership that is both authentic to you (therefore natural and sustainable) and also effective in the context in which you lead. Therefore, the 'best of you' is going to be authentically you, whilst also adapting your behaviour, as you need to, in order to be effective in leading your part of the health system. Within this, as we have also explored in Chapter 2, is an inherent tension to navigate, be authentic and adaptive!

I know a great psychotherapist, Jonathan, who says that everybody is unique, complex, fallible and valuable. I think this small sentence offers some real wisdom for leaders as a way to think of themselves and those they work with. First, if we are all *unique*, it would follow that our uniqueness needs to be one source for our authentic leadership. That if we are all *complex*, this requires an enquiry into all that makes us 'us' so we can be sure to be our best on the worst of days rather than leaving it to chance. Then understanding our own *fallibility* brings humility centre stage; that our perspective is valid but we need the humility to be open to being 'wrong' (and to then be interested when people think we are wrong, rather than defending our point). Then there is our value. Here Jonathan said that people nearly always agree with the first of his three words but not the fourth, that they are *valuable*. There is a lot to consider with this simple word – valuable, 'a thing of great worth'. If you were to say it in a sentence now, do you believe it at a deep level? Let's try it – say this to yourself now: 'I am valuable'. What do you notice as you ask this of yourself? To be authentic, we need to believe in our own value, that our contribution counts, that we are inherently valuable. At the same time, we need to believe it of those around us in our teams and organisations; they are also valuable, they count, they matter.

The authors of these chapters are faculty on programmes together and friends, and we share some core principles for leadership development that have influenced this book and certainly this chapter.

Self-awareness

Deep self-awareness is fundamental for a leader. If we are not aware of what drives our behaviour, we tend to project the limitations or frustrations we have internally onto other people and see them as the problem instead of recognising when an issue is our own. I recently worked with a leader who thought they had a performance issue with one of the team because of how much time this individual spent talking to colleagues as a part of getting on with the work. After a development session, the leader said:

> '*I thought I needed to have a performance conversation with this team member, but now I realise that what has been annoying me is firstly a different style that is actually a valid way of working which helps team dynamics. But I also now recognise that I am really judgemental if people don't work just as hard or in the same way as me; I tend to write them off as lazy or inconsiderate. But this is really my stuff I am projecting on to them, mainly because it is one of the things I don't feel free to do myself.*'

What a great moment of learning and growth!

Self-expression

Self-expression can be described as communicating so as to maximise the chance that you'll get meaningful outcomes out of every interaction. My colleagues writing this book share the view that, in some ways, you can only really lead through conversation; as you'll read in other chapters, the phrase 'leading one conversation at a time' reflects this and it is through conversation that a leader creates positive change. In a sense, the quality of a leader's communication really is the difference between a team turned round or not, patient care improving or diminishing, the real conversation happening in the room or a culture of corridor conversations and avoidance.

Self-possession

Drawing on this term from the writing of psychiatrist Norman Doidge (2007), this is the ability of a person to control their reactions and emotions even in stressful conditions. This is critical for a leader to be able to observe and make sense of situations around them, to notice their own emotional state, whilst in addition considering the group dynamic taking place. For example, a self-possessed leader is able to suspend being right in a discussion to bring out the necessary conversation and diverse perspectives. In our experience, it is critical for a leader to be aware of both the work that is going on and the group process that is happening at the same time. This is critical because of how profoundly a group dynamic will affect the way the work is delivered.

These three 'lenses' will appear in different ways throughout this chapter and shape the content of each section. I think it helps you to be aware of these and consider your own development against your awareness of yourself and others, your quality of communication, and your ability to read and work with the underlying group dynamics.

In January of 2015, I read the news about a man who was arrested for driving up the M6 motorway on a freezing cold morning without having cleared the ice off his windscreen. He had only scraped the size of a small envelope off the windscreen in front of his face, and was then driving at 90 mph. In a way, if a leader does not have self-awareness and self-possession, they are driving like this man – with seriously limited vision, which can be a risk to themselves and to others. The enquiry into how you can be the best of you on the worst of days is about getting the widest possible view of yourself and your context to be effective.

Who we are and how we are

Central to leadership is 'who we are' and 'how we are'. For example, leadership is deeply affected by 'who I am' because we are a product of our history, our childhood in particular. Our successes, failures, critical incidents and significant people shape who we are, greatly influence our perception of what leadership is, and what leadership is required in any given moment. 'How I am' is significant because our current state greatly affects how we perceive reality; our mood, energy levels, the impact of the previous meeting we were in all affect how we experience colleagues in the moment. For example, it affects whether we can cope with disagreement or see it as a challenge to our own authority. So much of our behaviour is not consciously processed; it is instinctive, run by the patterns laid down earlier in life. Therefore, developing as a leader requires an enquiry into everything that makes you 'you'.

I want to build on this framing; when working with another individual, it is important to be aware of 'who they are' and 'how they are'. The same factors apply; colleagues are shaped by their past and their reflexivity in the moment will be affected by their emotional state. Awareness of this can help a leader generate flexibility in the way they are working with someone, such as increasing the ability to look beyond the presenting behaviour in a colleague to what positive intent is behind it. This awareness is essential for sustaining healthy working relationships.

Then another layer I will add is that of dealing with work groups or teams – it matters 'who we are' and 'how we are' collectively. Here, the 'who we are' is important in order to understand the influences that come with a group dynamic. Then there is the question of 'who are we together?'. There is a need for clear context for teams; what your purpose is, what destination you are all working towards in terms of patient experience, innovation in service and performance outcomes. A clear sense of identity in a team, aligned with the purpose they are responsible for, helps create an internal accountability. This clarity of purpose becomes the line in the sand to which expectations are set and accountability for performance can be followed.

Then there is paying attention to 'how we are' as a group or team. It is normal for undercurrents of thinking and emotion to be occurring between team members. Differences in 'who we are and how we are' greatly affect a group dynamic; varying personalities and emotional needs can quickly lead to tension or frustration. Therefore, if a leader pays attention to how the team is collectively, they can help the group to notice these dynamics in themselves and others, taking more responsibility for the part they may each be playing and moving faster to the conversation that can help resolve an issue.

I heard a good example of a leader doing this well recently. A CCG Chief Officer described how she had noticed in her team meeting that the conversation was becoming a bit 'spiky' – emotionally heightened. She intervened simply by saying:

> '*I am noticing that there seems to be some tension in the conversation we are having. Let's pause and I would like each of you to say what is going on for you right now. I know that you're committed to the best outcome in the issue we are discussing, but if we don't pay attention to the emotion that is surfacing it'll get in the way of that commitment.*'

One of the team members on the receiving end of this described how helpful it was to have attention drawn to the group process. This enabled them to surface the deeper concerns, frustrations and hopes they had for this particular piece of work. With this intervention completed, they were able to continue with the work effectively, helped by a better understanding of each other's views and feelings regarding the situation.

The work of a leader is to focus on both the formal work and the underlying group processes. A Head of Midwifery described to me a ward in her hospital that had a reputation of poor behaviour amongst staff and multiple patient complaints for over a year. Her intervention to turn this around was to talk with each member of staff on and, off the record, ask them about what was going on for them and how they felt about the work, the ward dynamic and the ward's poor reputation. After the team was able to surface their feelings, process their frustrations, and hear that they had personal responsibility for changing the situation, the ward dynamic changed within days. So why had this not happened before? Previous interventions had not paid attention to the group process (how the staff felt and the dynamics they experienced), and so the situation remained. The relationships between people had been more significant than the individuals themselves. The Head of Midwifery acknowledged there is work to do still, but I see this as a great start and an act of leadership on her part.

I have mapped out these three dimensions of self, others and team in the diagram shown in Figure 5.1.

Take some time to think about these three levels of *who we are* and *how we are*. Make a note of how those dynamics play out in your colleagues, and the interaction between you, individuals and the team?

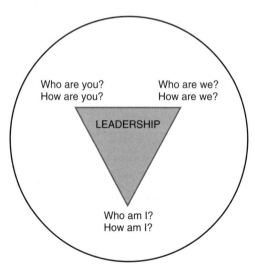

Figure 5.1 Dimensions of self.

needs to seek the best possible understanding of reality in order to solve a problem of patient flow or to bring about change between colleagues locked into disagreement and mistrust. Inherent within leadership is first being able to recognise that our opinion is an opinion rather than 'the truth'. Doing this enables a leader to hold their own point of view loosely enough to be able to fully hear and understand others' views. A major cause of conflict or misunderstanding that I experience working with leaders and teams is how certain people relate to their own opinion, combined with a lack of ability to see how someone else's viewpoint of the same situation could be valid.

I was recently working with a group of nurses and midwives when, mid programme, we took a coffee break and the group stood outside in the sunshine while I went for coffee. When I arrived back, an accident between a white van and a BMW had happened in front of the group. The group were split on their opinion about who was at fault. One half was convinced it was the van driver's fault and the other thought it was the BMW driver's fault. They were all utterly sure their perception of the situation was right and although the exchange of views was light-hearted, there was genuine disbelief that one group could possibly see it differently to the other. This conversation was polarised quickly to seeing people as those who are right and those who are wrong. In this case it had no consequence for the group, but so many conversations within the NHS and across the care system are of great consequence, and so a leader's ability to work beyond their own narrow perception to enable others to consider a bigger reality is fundamental. Once in this state, people tend to put their effort into defending the view they hold rather than exploring why someone else would see things so differently. You rarely see people persuaded through argument; the positions taken at the start tend to be better defended by the end, and relationships can easily be damaged in some way through this process. The 'so what' here is that a leader needs to see their perception as valid and mostly effective, and also to be particularly open and interested when people see the same situation differently to them. This requires holding your own point of view loosely enough to hear and enquire about alternative views. The leader then also needs to create a context in groups where others are able to do the same, to be open about their own perception and curious when other people's perception is different.

This is the first level of challenge and responsibility for a leader regarding perception. But there is a second level, namely, what we expect to happen is more likely to be what we then experience. We are playing a part in the behaviour of those around us.

Our perception has serious consequences. At one time I was working with two NHS organisational leadership teams who needed to work closely together but had deeply contrary opinions of each other. Team A thought team B were ineffective, had a victim mentality, always had an excuse for the lack of progress, and were never going to change. Team B thought team A were constantly serving their own agenda, pernicious in the way they dealt with others, and only used information that backed their own case to avoid helping with the challenges their organisation faced. Both teams were entirely convinced they were right – they had entirely different perceptions of reality that then drove their behaviour. Whatever seemed to happen, it was interpreted in a way that made more evidence for why their opinion was 'right'. Stories about incidents between the teams had become apocryphal. It did not matter if people were new to either team, they soon took on the shared opinion about the other team, and so on it went. In a sense, they were both right: they saw and interpreted data from a point of view that was already made up. This meant any data or incidents that were contrary to the team view would be twisted to reinforce the 'stock' perspective. This inability to understand situations from another person's or team's perspective was deeply divisive and had real consequences for patients. They were both playing a part in creating the reality they experienced. What they looked for, they found.

For a leader, the responsibility here is to check that they are not simply searching for the data and examples that reinforce the point of view they already hold about a person or situation. Conversations with others are essential to see a reality bigger than the one our own perception presents us. To do this requires a great capability in communication, and ability to self-possess.

This self-awareness around perception should not create faltering, hesitant leadership. A leader needs to know that perception is valid and also limited. You can trust it, and you need to test it, to be curious when people see things so differently and help teams engage in a reality bigger than the one they are defending.

Working with others

There is an old adage that people join organisations but leave bosses; often it is personal values and goals that influence which organisation we join, but it is a difficult or broken relationship with the boss that people often cite as the reason for leaving. As leadership requires engaging, enrolling or mobilising others to act effectively, effective dynamics between a leader and those they are working with is critical; it is particularly hard to enrol people if they are resistant to you.

When working with others there is a need for flexibility. How do you flex your style and approach to get the best out of others? The reality of leading is often messy, with conflict, disagreement, disruption to plans, interpersonal conflict and personality differences. This requires a leader to be flexible enough to hold the balance between being clear about what you want to see happen, and at the same time being able to adjust your style to help enrol those who are different to you.

With the goal of being the best of us on the worst of days, and for our enquiry into 'who we are' and 'how we are', understanding our own personality and the personality of those we work with is an essential element; this is what we are going to explore in this section.

You are likely to have explored aspects of your personality using psychometrics such as the Myers Briggs Type Indicator (MBTI®), Insights, 16PF or DISC. These (and many others) offer different but related insights into how your personality affects the way you see reality and how you are likely to go about your work and manage your relationships. These tools are descriptive. What is often missing is the 'why' we behave in the way we do. If we are aware of this part of personality formation, it can create a narrative that makes it easier to identify the patterns of behaviour in ourselves and others, and to see beyond the behaviour to the need that someone is trying to meet. I am going to share with you a 'causal' psychometric that can help you deepen awareness of yourself and of your colleagues. This psychometric has a range of different names depending on the phase of its development. The sources are the work of psychologist and author Alexander Lowen (1975), consultant and Visiting Fellow of Cranfield University Sandy Cotter (1996), psychologist and author Stephen M. Johnson (1994), and psychotherapist and author Ron Kurtz (2013).

If leadership requires being the best we can be whatever the circumstances, then key to this is to understand what drives us to be effective or ineffective at different times. In the table in Figure 5.2 there are six columns.

Column 1 is each personality numbered so it is easy to refer to a 'type', for example 'Elaine is primarily type 1 and 5'. Research suggests that we will have two or three of these personality influences that most show up in our behaviour and affect our perception of others.

Column 2 lists the names given to each type from a form of psychotherapy called the Hukomi Method. I am using these names because I think they capture something of the inherent tensions that are often behind the challenges leaders are facing in coaching or leadership development. We tend to understand that what is a strength of ours can also be a weakness when we are under pressure; in those moments we respond with unhelpful defences and a narrowing of our perspective. For example, people with the type 2 influence can be wonderful ambassadorial characters who can win people over as they are warm, playful and intelligent in conversation. The counter to this is that people with a strong type 2 influence can be overly dependent on the energy and drive of people around them, and when they perceive this is

Type	Name	Core need	How the 'core' need shows up	The 'best' of them	The 'worst' of them
1	Sensitive/ Analytical	Safety	I feel I have control or I feel threatened	- Principled - Quality thinking - Consistent - Analytical	- Over controlling - Judgemental - Explosive - Miss emotional information
2	Dependent/ Endearing	Attention	I feel connected to others or abandoned	- Relational - Ambassadorial - Playful - Sees emotional information	- Low energy - Blames others - Whining - Victim mind-set
3	Tough/ Generous	Power	I feel powerful or weakened (you are 'for' or 'against' me)	- Strategic - Breakthrough - Charismatic - Influential	- Ruthless - Dominating - Scheming - Creates own rules
4	Burdened/ Enduring	Approval	I feel approved of or punished	- Reliable - Hard working - Pastoral - Enduring	- Passive aggressive - Conflict avoidant - Resentful - Punishing
5	Industrious/ Over-focused	Success	I feel successful or a failure	- Outcome focused - Driven - Fairness/ Justice - Planning	- Insensitive - Inflexible - Over competitive - Hard driving

Figure 5.2 Five causal personality influences.

missing they can simply lack the drive to act effectively themselves and can be quite 'hard done to'.

Columns 3 and 4 identify the core 'need' that drives behaviour. There is a lot of theory behind this column, but the main premise from developmental psychology is that in the first six years of life we have five fundamental needs that change as we grow and our cognitive and emotional development progresses. For the first six months of life, when a baby has minimal cognitive processing ability, the primary developmental need is thought to be safety – that the child needs to experience a warm and welcoming environment. If the child then perceives this need is not met, then rather than this need blending into the background, it remains a primary need for the individual to function well as an adult – seeking safety through controlling their environment can be an adult version of this same babyhood need. A pattern of perceiving the world (remember the earlier content on perception) gets established where this personality type is unconsciously scanning for whether the environment is safe or not. This creates part of their contribution (great analytical and speedy thinking) and the behaviour that can undermine them when they feel threatened (overcontrolling or reactive). Hopefully, this will help you see the connection between the 'core need' becoming established and the next two columns, where the 'best' and 'least effective' behaviours play out.

Column 5 is the contribution each personality has to offer; in a sense this can be the best of them at the worst of times. It is the way someone with this personality influence tends to lead and contribute, where they naturally operate. The development challenge is how to demonstrate these behaviours more of the time. If you think this is a helpful way of thinking about learning for a leader, how might you be like this more of the time?

Column 6 is the point at which our core psychological need is not being met and so our more childlike defences show up. Describing these as the 'worst' of us is a way of saying that these are self-defeating defences that may help us be successful individually, but they are not effective in leadership as they represent a narrowing of perspective and operating often defensively out of our own version of reality. These behaviours become excluding of others and undermining for group effectiveness. The good news is that the more we develop self-awareness and self-possession, the less these needs drive our behaviour.

Here is a helpful piece of framing. First, we tend to have two or three of these personality types that most influence our behaviour. One of these influences may be more dominant than the others or they may be fairly equal. I know for myself I am predominantly type 5 with some 3 and 2. I have learnt in what context the 'worst' of me is likely to manifest and being aware of these patterns gives me more choice about how I can show up in those situations. The second piece of framing is that we are so much more complex than this simple chart. The longer I work in leadership development, the more I wonder at how remarkable and different we all are. At the same time, I see these patterns of 'best' and 'worst' at the heart of most leadership challenges. So paradoxically, if I had 10 leaders in front of me who were all type 4 and 5 personality influences, they would each be profoundly different from each other, and at the same time would share very similar type 4 and type 5 patterns of behaviour. Being able to identify in yourself and in others what core need is at work is a key that unlocks much deeper insight into why we behave in the ways we do. This understanding makes significantly more growth and change possible.

Here are two examples of a nurse and midwife leader learning about the impact of their personality on their leadership effectiveness.

Case study 1

I was working with a senior nurse who was struggling with delegation. She has a very strong need for control and success. As we discussed her challenge in delegating to her team members, I asked her what was important to her in terms of her leadership. She said that she needed to ensure that work was excellent, everything done to a high standard, ensuring strict adherence to the process and policy. I then asked what the opposite of all these things would be. She paused before she answered and then after about a minute said, 'well ... it would be anarchy'. When asked what it would feel like if situations were anarchy, as she perceived it, her response was 'fearful'. You can hear how she is making sense of the world; to her, situations are either in control and to the standards that she wanted, or they felt like anarchy. These are two extremes with no space between them. In reality, if a colleague of this leader did not deliver as she wanted and a deadline was missed, it would not suddenly be anarchy, probably no one would notice! However, to the leader it feels like this due to the strong influence of her type 1 personality. Growth for her as a leader was to experiment in giving away control, to change her view of 'either control or anarchy' and see a bigger reality than the one she is operating with.

Case study 2

In another example I was working recently in a group with one member – a senior midwife – who had a strong need for power (type 3). In the group conversation, she identified colleagues of hers as either being on board or against her. As the group asked questions as to what made someone against her, she identified that if people disagreed with her publicly or did not show her respect, she would see them as literally being against her. The group really helped her understand how she was defining people into 'for or against her' based upon her own emotional need to feel powerful and important. They were naming how she was making sense of the world. This leader needed to recognise the part that she was playing in the behaviour of those around her. There was a lovely moment of challenge as the group helped her face the choice of taking more responsibility for how she was experiencing the dynamics in her organisation. Again, we see here that the more we understand what drives our behaviour, the more choice it gives us about how we deploy our leadership, and how we could be the best of us regardless of how the day is.

Here is an exercise to help spot your personality influences and those of your colleagues.

1 Read through the table of the five personality influences (Figure 5.2) and identify the two or three that you think most influence you. We each tend to have a predominant two and sometimes three preferences. We are more complex than any simple model, but I do find these descriptors often get to the heart of how people are functioning.

2 Once you are clear on the two primary personality influences, consider when you are at your best and when you are your least effective, and in what conditions these behaviours manifest. The challenge here is to consider how you might become the best of you, whatever the circumstances. For example, if you spot some type 5 influence, do you notice your irritation when people are not as efficient or as driven as you? Do you oversimplify your assessment of people as competent or incompetent? Do you get frustrated when people want to engage socially at the start of a meeting when you want to be efficient and get on with the work? Noticing how you make sense of reality and make judgements about others is key to appreciating where your lens is too narrow – when you are only appreciative of others when they match your own preferences.

3 Next list your key team members or stakeholders that you want to focus on. Then consider which of the personality types they each demonstrate and when they tend to be more or less effective. Then consider the strategies you are using to engage with these people and how these may or may not be helping you influence them effectively. For example, if you are struggling with a working relationship with a very strong type 5 who is focused on outcomes, speed, efficiency and competence, but you are engaging very relationally and conversationally, they may perceive you as ineffective, time wasting or just irrelevant. The challenge here is how to adapt to their preference enough to have a real conversation that will help you make progress. You often find that once a sense of good working relationship is established then very different personalities to you will often become much more flexible as they perceive a sense of rapport and alignment with you.

4 Consider where you could draw on the personality preferences of your team or colleagues to get the best from them. How might you draw on their capabilities and preferences to help improve performance? Strong differences in personality are often the cause of conflict; disagreements, misunderstandings and a narrowing of perspective can easily occur when under pressure and when we are faced with people really different to ourselves. Leadership requires the ability to draw on the widest range of personality types possible – it is hard to enrol people if they are resistant to you, and so this flexibility is required in the way you work with difference.

I have worked in leadership development for 15 years and I am struck by how frequently these personality types are demonstrated, and at the same time how profoundly and wonderfully different every single person is. These descriptions should not define us but they are helpful as the more we understand about what drives our own and others' behaviour, the more choice this gives us in how we lead in different circumstances.

Setting teams up to perform well

I thought it would be helpful to explore what I do when a client asks me to help develop their team's performance. You can use the same thinking and templates as you consider the performance and effectiveness of teams and groups you work with.

There are two main frameworks on my mind. The first is about taking into context the purpose of this team in the wider organisation. This leads to enquiry into organisational culture, processes, workflows, measures of performance, how people are rewarded, how the organisation is structured. You'll know these things when you are in the organisation, but there is still real value in assessing them from time to time. How is the organisation set up in a way that could undermine you achieving the objectives you are accountable for? How might a wider organisational culture be driving behaviour in your team that could be undermining the standards you're trying to establish?

When meeting with a client and once I have an understanding of the broader organisational context, I then use the framework shown in Figure 5.3 to identify the developmental need. Improving team performance can require work on the agenda, developing better group dynamics, improving the approach to getting work done or development of individuals within the team. The 'four dimensions of team effectiveness' provide a framework for diagnosing team performance gaps and developing sustainable high performance in teams.

While the framework in Figure 5.3 is simple, ensuring that your team is strong in each of the four areas can really help to establish and sustain good performance. So let's think through each of these components of a high-performing team.

Quality of agenda

Quality of agenda is about ensuring that each team member is really clear about the work of the team. This can sound obvious, but I frequently find team members with very different understandings of the team's purpose. The purpose may be more obvious on a ward or a community team, but I think

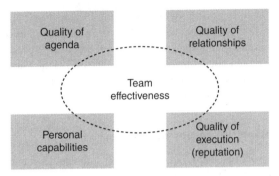

Figure 5.3 Effectiveness grid.

it's important not to assume that your team really understand the part they play in shaping the experience of patients and their contribution to the wider organisation.

Quality of agenda is about creating real intrinsic commitment to the shared agenda. The intrinsic buy-in here is critical; extrinsic commitment means people do things because they know they have to and because they are being watched or assessed. Intrinsic commitment means that people understand why something is required, they agree they have some responsibility for it happening well, and they then apply their energy and creativity towards getting the work done as well as possible. There is clearly a challenge to find time on a busy ward to have these conversations, but I would say you can't afford not to create the space for them. High levels of team participation in problem solving and idea creation are proven to increase engagement and responsibility among team members. Whether this is about understanding the current agenda, shorter-term initiatives or reviewing performance generally, conversations are key to getting a team aligned around the same work.

On one recent NHS Leadership Academy programme, a team leader nurse described how the involvement of her whole team, especially the healthcare assistants, with infection control had helped them dramatically reduce the incidence of infection. Her insight about what had made the difference was engaging her colleagues at the outset of the initiative: 'they all shaped the approaches for tackling this problem all the way through the initiative, you could tell that seeing the change through to the end mattered to them all'. One of the challenges sometimes directed at the NHS is that teams and departments work in isolation from each other. This is a common problem with any industry or organisation, but clearly with potentially such significant consequences in the health service. Engaging a team around their agenda and the part they are playing in the wider health system is critical for helping improve the quality of information, patient flow and collaboration across organisational boundaries.

Daniel Kahneman, in his book *Thinking Fast and Slow* (2011), refers to the problem of identification. This is that we identify so strongly with our department, function or role that we are suspicious of or less confident when accepting ideas or requests that come from a different part of the organisation. When you hear about team or department behaviour being particularly poor, you have to consider how this has happened so strongly and in isolation. If a team or department becomes isolated from the part they play in the wider organisation, the risk is that a self-referencing logic can become established which justifies practice that is not in the best service of the wider organisation. This is a strong case for the need to engage your teams and colleagues in the quality of your own agenda, in service of the wider agenda of patient care and compassion.

Quality of relationships

Given the nature of organisational life, with its conflicts, disagreements and constant change, combined with the emotive nature of the work in the health service, there is enormous pressure on staff and their relationships. Therefore it is essential to establish a quality of relationships that will work well under pressure, where the diversity in all senses strengthens collective performance, and enables a fulfilling teamwork experience, which is so fundamental for wellbeing in work.

Teams need to be able to create a dynamic through which they will create the best unfettered understanding of reality, and create effective conversations about how to tackle the complex issues and the 'wicked problems' that Keith Grint (2008) defines. A friend and leadership consultant, Todd Holzman, described how teams require a constructive tension where the real issues and challenges are named and discussed; what is un-discussable becomes discussable and, importantly, colleagues receive live feedback on performance and behaviour, regularly and consistently. Teams and leaders find this image of constructive tension helpful; too much tension and the focus is on the relationships and defensive discussion, too little tension and there is not enough attention on the issue at hand. Learning to create and navigate this constructive tension is central to the role of a leader. A leader's role is to create positive change and not simply manage the status quo.

I think one of the most helpful tools for establishing a quality of relationships is that from David Kantor's (2012) book *Reading the Room*. He identifies four action modes that show up in our conversation: Move, Oppose, Follow and Bystand. As a brief summary, a Move is to create movement and initiate. The Oppose is to bring correction or challenge. The Follow is supporting an idea or action. The Bystand, which can sound passive, is an essential role for teams to work well; it provides perspective and pays attention to the group process. Even with this short description, you can consider where your preference is out of these four actions. What pattern plays out in your team, where do you get stuck, what action mode is missing which you need to develop, how aware are team members of their preference? For example, I am working with a team that gets stuck with serial monologues; each person makes a point that is slightly different to the previous person's, and this goes on so time is taken up, the issue being discussed is no longer clear and often frustration builds. What this requires is first of all good bystanding to call out the pattern of a drifting conversation. It also needs those who oppose to say so, rather than avoiding opposing and making a new move. There is also a need for clear following; who does agree and is willing to support? I think you can see from this example that this is a framework well worth further exploration; it is so easily applicable in teamwork and is a fantastic tool for helping balance the contribution in a team and for creating the constructive tension required for great collective work.

One other factor in developing the quality of relationships is developing the personal connection. Clearly, to build relationships requires trust, and trust requires rapport for the relationship to get started. Therefore time spent getting to know who people are, what their interests are, and what connection you may have in common lays the foundations that trust can build on. It is harder to make snap defensive judgements about someone when you know a lot about what they have done, in work and personally, and what they value. Have you ever had the experience when you work with someone and find them irritating but then at some point you find out something about them which is fascinating, or about how they dealt with a very difficult situation, or just a really interesting experience they've had? Your attitude then changes, you have more grace and flexibility in the way you work with them.

So this is the challenge: how you take responsibility for creating a quality of relationships that works in service of the objectives for which you are accountable.

Quality of execution

Execution includes your planning, how you respond to organisational changes or performance pressures, how you collaborate with other departments, how you solve problems and work with both processes and culture to establish the performance you require. This is the everyday reality of ensuring high-quality and compassionate patient care.

Here, I want to offer you another piece of research that comes from Michael Tushman of Harvard Business School and Charles O'Reilly of

Stanford Graduate School of Business (1997). Although in the early days of your career you won't be engaged in setting the overall organisational strategy, this research is also relevant to leading a team or department. The story here is as follows: 'New strategy requires new execution; new strategy with old execution can give you the old strategy'. Mike and Charles have looked at what helps organisations succeed in the long term and how you can be more confident that the strategic objective will actually be delivered. One of the fundamental insights they offer is the need for congruence in execution.

When organisational change is being implemented, the attention is often on the organisational *hardware* (key activities and work processes, system enablement, formal organisation structure, clarity at interfaces, management systems and reward) and not enough on the *software* issues (people, skills, talent, behaviour, motivation, values and culture). This can result in new structures, metrics and processes, but the same behavioural and performance challenges remaining after the organisational change effort. A challenge with any organisational change effort is to get alignments between these different aspects of execution. Here's an example. I was running a session on culture change on the NHS Leadership Academy Nursing and Midwifery programme. One of the participants described the situation she had experienced when the 4-hour breach target was implemented. In the large general hospital where she worked, she went to meet with the head of the A&E department and noticed a new yellow line drawn on the floor. She asked her colleague what this was for, the colleague replied that it was to delineate one side being A&E and the other not. When pressed about this, her colleague answered that if the patient was about to breach the 4-hour rule, they could push them over the line in the trolley and that would mean they were out of A&E and then a breach would not occur.

This example exposes a lack of congruence in the implementation of the breach target. Here, a metric is established as a part of organisational hardware but not enough attention was paid to the culture of the A&E department with responsibility for meeting this target, who just find a work-around, or the patient flow and what would be blocking beds in the Medical Admissions Unit (MAU) and other pathways. In this case the metric seemed to be implemented in isolation without paying enough attention to the other aspects of execution, the lack of congruence resulting in ineffective execution.

I have seen many other examples of implementing change without considering the implications of both *hardware* and *software*. Even for small changes in a process, changes to how you measure performance or trying to establish different behaviours, considering how to get each aspect of organisational execution to reinforce the change you're seeking is really important. This definitely requires more work but this is a 'pre-work or re-work' moment – do the preparation work and you are more likely to see success, skip the preparation work and you are likely to be back into the conversation, working out how to try and embed the change again after it has failed to work at the first attempt.

Personal capabilities

This is the simplest part in one sense, ensuring you have people with the right skills and capabilities working on the team or project. But at the same time it can be challenging to develop the right behaviours that will in turn create the culture for 'how things are done around here'. I used to be a PE teacher in a secondary school and I had a mantra that would pop into my head when children were not behaving well: 'If you are not getting the behaviour you need for good learning then do something about it'. Simple but effective as a reminder to intervene even when there are small things going on that aren't quite right.

So for you it could be, 'Am I getting the behaviour we need for high quality and compassionate care? If not, do something about it'. One of the big killers of good culture is when someone gets good results but with poor behaviour. It is absolutely critical to hold these people to account, otherwise this can slowly unravel the standards you've set on your wards or across your patch. I once worked with a senior team in banking who were about to invest hundreds of thousands of pounds in training to develop their staff. But they were ignoring the strong and evident pattern of behaviour that people were promoting and lauding those who made lots of money for the bank but behaved appallingly. All that investment in training the leaders could be a waste of money because the real message employees get is, it doesn't matter how you behave, just make money. So your challenge is to identify the shortfall in both the skills and behaviour in colleagues, and have the conversations and put the plans in place to close these gaps.

So overall this is a helpful framework to diagnose current strengths and gaps in the way you help set the team up for success. It's really useful to come back and check against this framework from time to time, to use it with your team as a rationale for why you are doing certain things, especially investing in group conversations. I could hear you saying to your team as you show them this diagram, 'OK team, a great team is strong in all these four areas, let's have a conversation about where we are strong and where the gaps are; how we do more of what is good and how we deal with the shortfalls'?.

The power of humility

Humility is a vital virtue for leadership. This might not be something you associate with effective leaders, but I am convinced that demonstrating humility is central to great leadership. One of the reasons why humility is not normally associated with leadership is because humility is confused with thinking less of yourself or in some way a sign of weakness. The traditional view of leadership is about strength, certainty, asserting effectively. However, these are not mutually exclusive with humility. It takes enormous strength and at times courage to demonstrate humility. One reason why humility is not talked about much is that it's hard to say 'I'm humble' if you're humble! Psychological assessment of humility is tricky because the people who like to tell you how humble they are probably aren't that humble. So one way to describe this is that humility is not thinking less of yourself but thinking of yourself less. Humility is important because it is about giving space for others to flourish, which is critical in leadership.

If you review the content of this chapter, there are aspects of humility required in each of the behaviours described. For example, to acknowledge that much of your behaviour is driven by the unconscious and to have a willingness to acknowledge that your point of view is just that, your point of view, requires humility. When it comes to personality, to recognise that your perception of others is deeply coloured by your own preferences also requires humility. I worked with a team recently and after the development session, the team leader said that he had thought he had a performance issue with one of the team, but now after learning about his own personality, he realised that the person in question was simply someone with a different personality. The realisation that the team leader had a lack of flexibility because he found the other team member's personality annoying is a pretty important insight. It enabled him to appreciate the contribution this person's personality offered the team, while also increasing awareness of his own limits in flexibility when it came to working with different people. In this case I think this is humility at work – this is a virtue in his character that strengthens his leadership.

Thinking back to the earlier discussion about leadership being about 'who we are and how we are', it requires humility to appreciate how profoundly these two things affect our experience of reality. As the author Rick Hanson (2013) writes, 'Thoughts are like rumours, sometimes they are true'; we need humility about our perception of reality. Thinking about setting the team up to work well, there is humility in recognising that people see things that we don't see and recognising the need for alternative views to get a better understanding of what might really be happening. Particularly if you need to admit you were wrong about something.

I was once asked by a client in a global sportswear brand to come and help with her team. The briefing was different from normal – she said, 'I'm stuck, my team are dysfunctional and I don't know what to do. I'm an experienced and successful leader but for some reason I can't seem to make progress in the way we work together'. It was so refreshing to hear a very senior leader say things just how they were; there was courage in addressing the issues in this way. The act of humility here was to take off the mask of perfection in favour of facing this reality. There is a general expectation that a leader's communication and interaction will be slick, positive and effective. But the gift of humility here is to be less James Bond smooth than I know I like to portray. Organisational life and leadership are usually pretty messy, particularly when the pressure is on. There's a lovely saying attributed to Edwin Friedman, and quoted by the author Susan Scott in her book *Fierce Conversations* (2002): 'The person who can most accurately describe reality without laying blame will emerge as the leader'. See, the power of humility!

Another area where humility plays a significant part is effective group communication. I mentioned in the introduction that we think that communication is the primary tool of a leader; it is through conversation that a leader deploys their influence to create positive change. When it comes to group conversation, much of the time is spent in discussion that could be more effective. In his book *Dialogue and The Art of Thinking Together*, William Isaacs (1999) writes about how the word 'discussion' comes from the origin of 'percussion' – which means to bang together – versus dialogue, which means thinking together. This definition alone is helpful for identifying the fundamental flaw in discussion. I'm sure you have experienced plenty of conversations that were ineffective, where people were competing for airtime. What I think is most missing from these situations is humility.

In a conversation, this looks like people balancing both advocacy and enquiry as Jamie and Philippa have written about in Chapter 7. We often have the impulse to drive home our point of view when people disagree, but in that moment, if we can instead move to enquiry to understand why people see things differently from us, then learning can continue. Have you noticed how it feels like a conversation starts to stall as points of view get traded across the table. In that moment of competing to have your point of view heard, learning is not taking place and this can establish an unhealthy dynamic of those who are included or excluded within the group. If you want to find agreement, find the disagreement in the room first and work through it meaningfully. This requires the humility to hold on to your perspective lightly, even if you're convinced about it, particularly when you're passionate about the subject and the pressure is on.

A friend of mine mentioned he was reading a book called *Humble Enquiry* by Edgar Schein (2013). Schein is a well-known author of major texts on organisational culture and change, and his latest book is about, in his words, the gentle art of asking instead of telling. I think there is wisdom in this.

To sum up why I see humility as a core virtue of effective leadership, I have three points. First, humility is required to recognise that perception is unique to each person and that we will all have blind spots. Second, humility is immensely effective in helping create a context in which others can be heard and contribute. Remember the earlier definition of humility as giving space for others to flourish. The third reason why I think humility is so important in leadership is that it enables you and your colleagues to operate from a greater reality than the one you are hooked into. Humility is a virtue that acts like a gateway into more effective personal and collective leadership.

This reminds me of a senior NHS leader who met with me at a time of incredible pressure in the large hospital where she worked. She was hooked into a very difficult and negative view of the reality she was facing in her role, which was causing her to feel enormously stressed and at risk. A few hours later when she left our meeting, she was much more at peace and had a new plan of attack. This was not brilliance on my part but rather that, between us, we simply managed to gain sight of a bigger sense of reality than the one she was hooked into when she arrived.

The challenge is, how do you develop leadership? I'm so humble so let me tell you how to do this! Ah yes, it does not work quite like that. But I do think that the three practices can help: holding your own point of view loosely so you can enquire effectively into why other people see things differently; taking responsibility for how you experience everything; conducting rigorous investigation into your interior life to understand more of who you are and how you are.

References

Cotter, S. (1996) Using bioenergetics to develop managers. *Journal of Management Development*, 15(3), 8–16.

Doidge, N. (2007) *The Brain That Changes Itself*. New York: Penguin Books.

Fromm, E. (1976) *To Have Or To Be? The nature of the psyche*. New York: Harper and Row.

Grint, K. (2008) Wicked problems and clumsy solutions: the role of leadership. *Clinical Leader*, 1(2).

Hanson, R. (2013) *Hardwiring Happiness*. London: Ebury Press.

Isaacs, W. (1999) *Dialogue and The Art of Thinking Together*. New York: Random House.

Chapter 6 **Influencing with integrity**

Louisa Hardman

If nurse leadership is about enrolling others to maintain and improve patient experience then influencing lies at its heart. Without influence, great ideas never see the light of day, services never improve and frustration replaces innovation. Your ability to influence really can enhance care and save lives. This chapter will show you how.

Getting started

Before we start, please take a moment to identify:
- who you want to influence about what
- what gives you the right to do so

Understanding influence

It's an interesting first exercise this one, isn't it? As well as raising all kinds of questions about authority and confidence, it also prompts us to ask what we mean by influencing in the first place. It turns out that this is an important question, primarily because many of us have qualms about being manipulative. So, before we do anything else, let's first define our terms.

According to the *Oxford English Dictionary*, influencing means 'the capacity to have an effect on the character, development or behaviour of someone'. Of course, we all do that all of the time, even when we don't intend to, don't we? If you've ever received 360° feedback then you'll be aware that even how we enter a room and greet people can have a significant impact on their mood. What's different about the kind of influencing that we're talking about

How to be a Nurse or Midwife Leader, First Edition.
Edited by David Ashton, Jamie Ripman and Philippa Williams.
© 2017 John Wiley & Sons, Ltd. Published 2017 by John Wiley & Sons, Ltd.

here is that you *intend* to have a particular impact. You want to engage others to achieve a specified service improvement, for example. This is what makes some people uncomfortable as they then wonder if they are *manipulating* rather than *influencing*.

So, what's the difference? Well, rather a lot as it turns out. Again, let's look at the *Oxford English Dictionary*, which defines manipulation as 'handling or controlling a person or situation cleverly or unscrupulously'. We're certainly not doing the 'unscrupulous' bit though it's true that we may need to be 'clever' in mobilising change. The main differences probably lie in your openness about your intentions and the morality of the collective benefit that you're after. But you need to make your peace with the distinction as if you don't feel comfortable about influencing, then you're not likely to work at it.

Returning to our first exercise, the second question usually also needs initial and continuing work, particularly as you meet the inevitable resistance along the way. What gives you the right to influence? Why should anyone follow you? How can you keep on going when so many around you disagree?

These questions point to the importance of the first of the six aspects of effective influencing we'll work through in this chapter: how do you manage your state of mind?

Managing your state

Influencing is a process, it takes time and you will usually encounter resistance and even ridicule before you achieve success. Consequently, very much as we explored in Chapter 3, you will need to manage your resilience in order to persist and bolster your confidence to even begin. Anne Dickson (1982) has a wonderful phrase to describe how we respond to criticism and put-downs: the 'crumple button'. We know when it's been pushed as we collapse and shrink into defensiveness and negative feelings even though the catalyst may be just a word, tone, phrase or look. You need to prepare for yours being pushed as, if you really care about what you're trying to achieve, it likely will be. Do you know what presses your crumple button? Uncomfortable as it may be to think about this, it really helps to know as then you can anticipate rather than be floored by it.

More broadly, you're unlikely to even start trying to influence or, if you do so, you may find yourself being quite half-hearted about it, unless you're fully confident about the importance of what you're doing. For a moment, then, think again about the questions in the exercise above, 'who do you want to influence about what?' and then consider 'what gives you the right' to seek to change your colleagues' thinking and practice? There are many things that may come to mind so let's look at a few of them. It's useful to remind yourself about these 'rights' both at the outset and throughout your influencing endeavour.

Maybe you have practical expertise borne of experience and education so that you know and understand what others don't? Or your work may give you a special insight into patient impact that others can't possibly share? You possibly have access to information from your networks and connections that others may not be aware of? Or your networks may be the reason that you're the right person to be influencing for change as you are so widely connected that you can easily spread an idea? Whichever it is, anchor it into your thinking so that you can recall your 'right' and revive your commitment.

Even if none of these apply, there is something else. Maybe you just have a great idea, an idea that no-one else has thought of or developed and, as Victor Hugo says, 'all the forces in the world are not so powerful as an idea whose time has come'. So, you need to be the voice of your idea, to be confident for your idea even if not for yourself. Equally, the thought of your being the voice of yet unrealised patient benefit can be a wonderfully enabling resource when all the voices around you are unsupportive. Think of that future patient looking you in the eye rather than being dissuaded by the gaze of a reluctant colleague.

Stephen, a Lead Nurse and Deputy Director of Infection Prevention and Control, was becoming increasingly concerned by his colleagues' apparent reluctance to discuss, let alone consider improving, their infection control protocols despite notable increases in catheter-associated urinary tract infections. Having always previously influenced through friendly conversation using facts and data, Stephen was at an impasse as he did not want to offend his colleagues or cause conflict yet knew that he had to be more forceful:

> *'I imagined myself explaining to a future patient that their infection was caused by our practice which made me more assertive with my team. Infection rates are now going down because I was bold for my patients, not for myself.'*

Usually, strengthening confidence on the inside translates into confidence on the outside but sometimes we need a reminder about how to embody our ideas so that they stand their best chance of being convincing.

Managing your stance

This aspect is intimately linked to the topic we explored in Chapter 2. Here is how it links to our ability to influence. I was recently working with two directors from the National Theatre on powerful communications. They usefully started the seminar with a reminder about Professor Mehrabian's work (1971) on the importance of congruence between words, tone and body language. Interesting, isn't it, that most of us tend to prepare the content of what we hope to say and give much less, if any, attention to either our state or our tone of voice and body language? Yet, if someone doesn't look and sound like what they are saying is important, then are we convinced? Probably not, maybe even to the tune of Mehrabian's research, which suggests that our content counts for a mere 7% of our appeal, with congruent tone claiming 38% and our overall demeanour topping the scale with 55%.

So, before you enter the meeting room, spend some time working through Chapter 2 and definitely watch the now famous Amy Cuddy TED Talk 'Your Body Language Shapes Who You Are'. Those 'power poses' really work!

In this chapter, I would like to emphasise the importance of tone. I've noticed that many nursing colleagues often sound like they are asking for permission rather than making a proposal simply because their tone of voice ascends at the end of a sentence. Try it – ask a question now as you're reading this, something irrelevant though tempting like 'Would you like a cup of tea?'. Did you hear how your tone lifted to create a question? Now drop the questioning tone and repeat the question. Did you notice how it now sounds like you're making a statement? Imagine what a difference it makes if you think you're emphatically stating the importance of a service innovation and your audience hear you asking their permission! Your idea deserves a confident tone.

Similarly, the excellence of your idea can easily be overshadowed by the diffidence of your body language. So ask yourself how you can use your body language to be the best possible vehicle for your proposal. You may feel more or less confident as a person but this isn't about you – you're embodying your idea and, if it's a good one, then it needs you to look strong and sure. Again, the National Theatre directors had a memorable approach to working stance, the idea of a behavioural status gauge. If you imagine that your physical posture can be changed by the twist of a dial from one to ten, where are you? If your posture says 'two' and your idea needs an 'eight' then you need to dial yourself up to scale!

The Strozzi Institute's work on Somatic Coaching (Strozzi-Heckler, 2014) emphasises the importance of posture for influence and looks at three dimensions: standing tall for dignity, wide for social space and deep for gravitas. Having regularly used this myself, I can vouch for its benefits, particularly on the pace of delivery, which so often speeds up when we become anxious! So stand up for your suggestion while you're waiting for others to join you.

Managing your style of engagement

Before we unpack the idea of influencing style, I would ask you to imagine yourself influencing somebody you anticipate finding difficult to convince. In your mind's eye, imagine how you'll begin, what they'll say, how you'll respond and how you're likely to feel. Now let me ask you … did you ask them any questions about their perspective or reluctance?

Interesting, isn't it? Most of us don't ask anywhere near enough questions when we're seeking to influence, especially when we anticipate meeting someone who is unlikely to support us. Instead, we tend to say more, speak faster and strengthen our case. Yet influencing isn't about winning an argument nor about defeating the opposition; it's about engaging colleagues' interest and inclination so that they will work with us to realise an idea. Whilst we *know* this, the moment we start to *feel* defensive we forget and when we feel defensive we tend to insist more stridently and, ironically, appear weaker, indicating that our arguments are flawed. Put simply, defensiveness is the enemy of influence and curiosity is its antidote.

This is exactly what John Heron (2001) describes in his work on helping styles, which distinguishes Push styles from Pull approaches (Figure 6.1). Pushing is mostly about authoritatively persuading with facts and logic whilst Pulling emphasises asking questions and working with the emotions. Thinking back to your imagined conversation, which style did you tend to use and did you ask enough or any questions? For example, imagine that you want to introduce innovations in older people's services. The kinds of questions you could ask include the following.

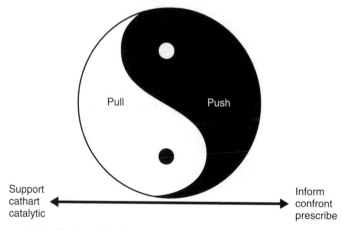

Figure 6.1 Facilitative and authoritative approaches.

- I'd like to tell you about my ideas for improving older people's services. Before I say more, I'm very interested to understand your perspective and interest in this area.
- I anticipate that we may have different starting points based on our varied experiences of older people's services. What are your interests and concerns about the current situation?

It is clearly *so* useful to understand your colleague's thinking. Not only do you indicate interest in them, you also begin to understand how you can frame your suggestions around their primary concerns and reservations. We will build on this in Chapter 7 when we look at the concept of blame-free conversations.

An equally powerful place for questions is during a conversation when you start to feel pressurised, challenged or overwhelmed. As counterintuitive as this sounds, asking a question when you feel in the grip of the adrenaline response can change the whole direction of a discussion. Again, imagine you're in the middle of a presentation on your thinking and the group is generally resistant to your suggestions. You could say:

- The points you're making (summarise them) are important. In your view, how could we strengthen the idea to reflect your concerns?
- Your reactions indicate that there are issues I've not considered. I'd like to pause to make sure we all have a full appreciation of our shared interests and reservations.
- If you could suggest one thing to strengthen this idea, what would it be?

A good question helps to reveal myriad important interests and, remember, it is quite unlikely that you'll have thought of everything. So, you could helpfully see criticism as offering you the insight to strengthen your thinking.

A similarly counterintuitive yet powerful approach is the idea of influencing by describing the problem rather than just your solution. If you take ownership of the problem and develop a solution, then you offer your colleagues the relatively limited scope of either agreeing or disagreeing with your suggestion. If, on the other hand, your influence starts with agreeing the problem that you face together then you have engaged colleagues at a much deeper and more personal level – in the 'why' and not just the 'what' This is precisely what Roger Fisher and William Ury talk about in their seminal book *Getting To Yes* (2012), researched and applied in national and international peace negotiations, such as Camp David. For them, there are four essential principles of effective negotiation which I find also apply to influencing.

- Focus on interests not positions.
- Separate the people from the problem.
- Invent options for mutual gain.
- Insist on using objective criteria.

If you would like to understand these principles in more depth then I thoroughly recommend reading their book.

As we really think about these four principles, what becomes clear is that they take us straight back to Heron's Push/Pull idea by reinforcing the importance of building strong relationships (focus on interests not positions, separate the people from the problem, invent options for mutual gain) and powerfully expressing a strong case for change (insist on using objective criteria) in a 3:1 ratio. If I observed you, would I see this 3:1 ratio as you attempt to enrol your colleagues? This, of course, is a question of context and skill so let's look at this in more detail so that you can rebalance your ratio!

Influencing with skill

Some years ago I came across an image describing the different psychological levels at which influence can work (Figure 6.2).

As you can see, the first two restate the 3:1 ratio in a different way; we need to be convincing (head) but also need to make people care (heart) about our recommendations. Only then will our colleagues be inclined to find the commitment to develop or invest their capability. Patient stories are, of course, a clear illustration of the influential power of creating a human connection that makes us feel. In fact, I've just come away from a conversation with a colleague who, as a hospital complaints manager, had prepared a comprehensive action plan to discuss with the family of an elderly patient who had died prematurely because of a drugs error. This is a very compassionate manager who only put her action plan away and allowed herself to feel the impact of the family experience when they sat a portrait-sized picture of the patient on the table. Similarly, it's helpful to ask ourselves how we can make our colleagues really care about an issue. As the model indicates, creating an emotional impact is critical if we are genuinely going to mobilise commitment and action. Carmine Gallo's recent book *Talk Like TED* (2014) builds on this by showing that the most popular TED talks are those delivered by speakers

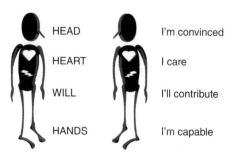

Figure 6.2 Head and heart.

who show real feeling and passion for their topic. In fact, 65% of the impact of the talks was attributed to this with a meagre 25% locating in the argument and 10% in the credibility of the person delivering.

There are many popular descriptions of influencing skills available. Fiona Dent's excellent book on influencing (Dent and Brent, 2010) and Robert Cialdini's (2007) descriptions are both worth checking out if you want to read further. With these frameworks in mind, I ran a series of workshops on the NHS Leadership Academy's Nursing and Midwifery programmes and found that the more relevant and important influencing skills to develop for participants were quite particular to the nursing community in a caring context. So, I have developed a new model of influencing skills to reflect these workshop conversations. Bearing in mind our initial question 'who do you want to influence about what?', let's explore these in some depth so that you can work out your influencing strengths, areas for development and potential approaches to achieve your current influencing agenda.

First of all, the influencing model for nurse leadership is as follows, presented as a ladder to represent the order in which the skills need to be used (Figure 6.3). This ordering also reflects earlier points, emphasising the importance of moving from Pull to Push styles (see Figure 6.1).

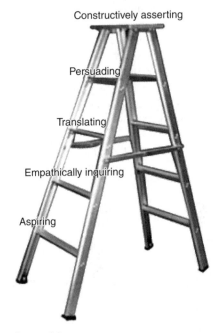

Constructively asserting

Persuading

Translating

Empathically inquiring

Aspiring

Figure 6.3 Influencing model.

Aspiring

We start with aspiring because you do; all influence starts with the end in mind. Some years ago I worked with Jocelyn Cornwell to introduce the Hospital Pathways/Point of Care methodology into the UK health system. This approach began with nurses and clinicians walking the patient journey with them – literally shadowing their experience. The impact of taking up the patient perspective was profound: the experience of waiting, interactions, the caring environment, the team dynamic, treatment handovers all being acutely felt, maybe for the first time. Such profoundly felt experience almost inevitably led to passionate aspirations for improvement, each of which was keenly held. The Point of Care approach attaches great significance to this stage of change and, at the time I was involved, brought teams together from across the UK to present and explore each other's aspirations through a storyboard approach. The effect of this was to create a clear confidence in and commitment to realise these aspirations in practice.

There was also very practical benefit, as the conference required participants to describe briefly their aspiration so that colleagues could comment and build on the ideas. Having to articulate ambitions to an experienced and insightful peer group meant that these nurse leaders had to ask themselves some important and sometimes uncomfortable questions, such as:

- How do I want patients to experience care under my leadership?
- What do I want patients to be saying, feeling, seeing and hearing about their care?
- What's the gap that I need to close to achieve this?

I commend these questions to you, alongside the discipline of producing a short summary of your aspiration. Your summary could take the form of a brief 'elevator pitch' (for which, see resources on Stanford University's website: www.stanford.edu), maybe using a simple framework such as:

- A – Aspiration: What's my aspiration?
- B – Benefits: What will the benefits of achieving this be?
- C – Consequences: What are the risks and implications of not doing this?

During the workshops, I noticed that articulating an aspiration was very challenging for people for various reasons. Some felt uncomfortably impractical about just having an aspiration whilst others felt that aspiration verged on arrogance and egotism. If any of these reactions resonate with you then please remember that nothing happens without a dream (history might have been different had Martin Luther King said 'I have a project'!) and that this aspiration is not about you or for you – it is *through* you. You are the voice of future patient experience that remains silent unless you find your tongue.

> • How do you rate yourself out of 10 on aspiration as a skill?
> • How can you use this to benefit your current influencing agenda?

Empathic inquiring

Earlier in the chapter, we noticed how rare it is to ask questions when you're *certain* that you're right and *passionate* about the change you're seeking to introduce; we also recognised that, unless you ask questions – even when feeling protective, indignant and defensive – then you can't tailor your stance to your audience. However, I term this skill 'empathic inquiry' as it goes beyond asking ordinary questions and traditional active listening and involves you engaging at a different level of openness, even when your inclination is to disagree.

So, first of all, empathic inquiry is an attitude in which you bring compassion to your interaction with colleagues. While this mindset may be our natural orientation with patients, it is often relatively absent with co-workers! We can nurture this by asking ourselves questions to ensure we stand in their shoes and see their world from their perspective. What pressures are they currently under? Who and what may be causing them concern? Why should they be interested in your suggestions? Why might they not agree with you?

Secondly, empathic inquiry is about asking significant questions with genuine curiosity. A test question for this orientation is to imagine that an important colleague disagrees with you and then ask yourself, how might they be right? Because they may be and their perspective could add the essential ingredient that ensures your proposal flies – but if you're not genuinely open to it and actively searching it out then you will miss the nugget and your notion will flounder. This, of course, is the trick – to listen as if your idea depended on it, as if this perspective will be the finishing touch.

Which means that you're also asking a different kind of question. Fisher and Ury (2012) talk about exploring interests, not positions, and that's exactly what you're doing here. Rather than asking a question like 'what do you think about the proposal for accelerated discharge?', you are asking 'what are your priority concerns about bed management?'. Rather than asking 'what are your reservations about our plans for a restructure?', you are asking 'what criteria should inform any restructure?'. Being broader, these kinds of questions are inherently more interesting and serve to build engagement with you even before they enhance engagement with your idea.

> • How do you rate yourself out of 10 on empathic inquiry as a skill?
> • How can you use this to benefit your current influencing agenda?

We'll come back to this when we explore blame-free inquiry in Chapter 7.

Translating

This is the critical and often missing linking skill between empathic inquiry and persuasion because it shows your audience that you understand and respect their perspective. Maybe even more importantly, you answer the questions that most proposals assume: what does this mean for me, to me; how does this benefit me; what advantage does this bring; how does this contribute to managing my workload, concerns, pressures or ambitions?

So, for example, let's say that you are wanting to introduce a new shift pattern to a group of colleagues who have expressed that they are concerned about damaging team morale. In your response, you might describe how the earlier pattern impacted morale and describe how the new approach will build on this, so that morale will be sustained but in new ways. The key here is that you adapt your arguments to that particular audience's priority interests.

Underuse of the skill of translating explains why the introduction of change can go so very wrong right at the outset. Empathic inquiry often reveals that colleagues accept the need for change whilst also needing to know that their earlier efforts have been worthwhile. Yet frequently, new proposals are presented in such a way that they suggest all previous practice has been faulty, so immediately causing resistance and resentment. In addition, the emphasis on change suggests that *everything* is changing and nothing remaining constant. Thoughtful use of the skill of translating would allow us to emphasise what will remain the same, alongside what will change whilst confirming that the change builds on earlier successes.

- How do you rate yourself out of 10 on translating as a skill?
- How can you use this to benefit your current influencing agenda?

Persuading

Translating clarifies the interests, concerns and therefore arguments that matter to your audience. You then need to pull everything together to ensure that you are offering a compelling case and this is the art of persuasion.

To illustrate this, I have recently been working with a group of senior nurses seeking to change orthopaedic care. When we came together to hear the proposals they had prepared for engaging senior colleagues, the majority of their content was an analysis of the problem. Now, no matter how compelling the myriad causes of an issue, we agreed that this approach would secure no further funding, for several reasons. Let's look at these reasons and how they apply to you.

The first was that they simply said far too much, making it easy to switch off and miss the main point. As you'll have read in Chapter 4, Blaise Pascale said 'If I had more time, I would have written a shorter letter'; brevity takes preparation and therefore time. Saying less brings emphasis and authority to your delivery.

The second reason was that they had not used translating emphatically enough to adjust the data to their audience's interests and concerns. Being persuasive doesn't mean saying everything, just making the most important points for this particular group of people. The more personally relevant you make your arguments, the more naturally engaging you are. Useful questions to guide your preparation include:

• Why might this particular group be interested in or opposed to my suggestions?
• What does my proposal mean for this audience in practice?

The third point was that their reasoning preceded their suggestions. Although this is counterintuitive, it is always more powerful to make a clear proposal and then clarify the rationale. Doing this in reverse means that if your audience disagrees with *any one* of your reasons then they automatically reject your idea. Let's look at this with a simple, day-to-day example.

Example A

I'm thirsty and haven't had my necessary fluid intake today. I also haven't seen many of my colleagues this morning. In addition, I need a break from all this hard work. What's more, I'm down on flavonoids. So would you please show me where the kitchen is so that I can make myself a cup of tea?

Example B

Would you please show me where the kitchen is so that I can make myself a cup of tea? I'm thirsty and need a break to be able to do my best work.

Quaintly eccentric though Example A is, it is neither as clear nor engaging as Example B. Yet this is how we often write or speak when we need to influence others.

You'll also have noticed the fourth reason in this last example – which is to offer no more than three good, strong reasons to back up your proposals. Why? Well, how many of the reasons given in Example A did you actually remember? And this is the point; research into short-term memory repeatedly shows that we easily remember three items. So make your persuasion easy for your colleagues to remember.

Even then, there are limits to persuasion. Drawing from your empathic inquiry and translation, persuasion is essentially offering your audience clear rational reasons for change which speak to their interests. There are times when this will not be enough and you will need to use our fifth influencing skill, assertion.

- How do you rate yourself out of 10 on persuading as a skill?
- How can you use this to benefit your current influencing agenda?

Constructive assertion

I find that helping professionals are often constitutionally uncomfortable about using assertion, feeling that it equates to being selfish, arrogant or egotistic. The result is often saying 'yes' to more and more, feeling put upon (and maybe even slightly resentful) until one of two things happens: either an outburst (at home or work – family often bear the brunt of unexpressed feelings at work) or exhaustion from trying to be everything to everyone. Recognise either of these? If you do, then influencing generally and assertion specifically will be extremely beneficial and not only when you're seeking to influence a change in practice.

At least some of this disinclination probably arises from the fact that assertion is confused with aggression. So let's be clear about the difference. Aggression is behaviour that pursues self-interest. When a colleague shouts, does not listen or carries on doing what they've always done because it is easier for or benefits them, then that's aggression. Assertion is different. It channels emotion into thoughtful, respectful expression in pursuit of constructive action. Every person who has ever spoken out for patient safety will have used assertion and all the new Freedom to Speak Up Guardians will need to become friends with it (see more information about this role on www.cqc. org.uk). In other words, it is an approach that is essentially helpful, which is why I have called this skill constructive assertion, to emphasise the point.

What, then, is different about constructive assertion? Compared with all the other skills, it involves more individual disclosure and leads to you making a personal request of another person. Whilst your request will be carefully calibrated, it remains unusual for us to request something of another person in a professional context on the basis of our personal feelings, preferences or reactions. How often do you find yourself saying anything like the following and would it be useful if you did?

- I'm feeling vexed about this meeting over-running and would like us to start on time in future.
- I notice that our conversations often become critical rather than constructive and would like us to focus on what we can rather than can't do from now on.

These statements are clear and powerful, partly because it is impossible for another person to argue with how you're feeling, even if they don't feel the same way. This, combined with the fact that your request is so clearly beneficial to all, is what characterises constructive assertion.

> • Before you read on, please take some time now to think of past situations you left regretting having said nothing.
> • Using the structure of (a) statement of feeling leading to (b) request, what could you have said?

'I was starting to feel really demotivated,' said Georgia, Head of Midwifery and Clinical Services. *'My new Director of Nursing was under a lot of pressure which was impacting her leadership style. We would discuss problems and agree clear timescales for actions. Before long, she would either have asked for an update, resolved the issue herself or changed her mind. I didn't feel trusted and questioned my competence.'*

Georgia explained that she would normally have internalised the issue without saying anything, allowing her frustration to build up before probably making an unhelpful comment. This time, she resolved to use the feeling–request structure preventatively, before the situation deteriorated. Her timing wasn't perfect – a rushed corridor conversation – but nonetheless Georgia took the opportunity to say 'I feel that you don't trust me when you check on my work so regularly. Can we discuss how we work together?'.

Georgia reports that this was a delicate turning point and that her Director of Nursing hadn't realised the impact of her behaviour. It created more mutual respect and new working arrangements.

Beyond this approach, constructive assertion can be strengthened as needs be by mentioning what will happen if your request is not followed. Though this is clearly more emphatic, it remains respectful and helpful because you are citing consequences of importance to your colleague/s and inherently seeking a positive outcome.

Developed by Sheppard Moscow to support leaders to influence without hierarchical authority, the elements of this approach are as follows.

1 Say what you like.
2 Say what you don't like.
3 Say what you want.
4 Say what will happen if this doesn't happen.
5 And what will happen if it does.

Source: Reproduced with permission of Sheppard Moscow LLP

Taken together, this offers a tried and tested way of approaching the genuine challenge of saying a purposeful 'no' when the many requests coming your way are deflecting you from important priorities.

Trevor, Interim Associate Director of Nursing, was quickly becoming overwhelmed with the deluge of requests coming his way. Being 'interim' meant that he was trying to prove himself by being everything to everybody. He wanted the substantive role but was beginning to think that this acting arrangement seemed like the longest interview he would ever have. What was worse, he was beginning to let people down; saying 'yes' to everything was influencing perceptions of his reliability, his responsiveness and his professionalism. He had to do something.

He decided to use the Five Step framework with his Director of Nursing and recalls saying something like:

1 *I'm really enjoying the scope of this new role.*
2 *Though, being new and keen, I am finding that everyone expects me to do everything.*
3 *So, what I've decided to do is to focus on the critical priorities and would like your support to confirm what these are.*
4 *I'm worried that if I don't do this then we'll all be increasingly busy but achieving less for patient care.*
5 *But, with our alignment and focus, I think that I can make some important improvements during my interim role.*

We offered this framework on the nurse leadership programmes and it proved instantly popular and enduringly useful. There were interesting conversations about points (4) and (5) seeming maybe punitive and even aggressive, which would be the case if you weren't pointing to consequences that your colleague cares about. For example, you are *not* saying to a consultant colleague 'I respect your aim to improve the service but stop interrupting patient mealtimes or I'll report you to the Medical Director'. You are more likely to be saying 'I respect your aim to improve the service though I'm less comfortable with the way you're approaching my nurse colleagues. So, let's spend some time looking at how we can work together on improving patient care. If we don't, I'm worried that your good ideas won't gain traction. If we do then I'm confident we will be able to implement significant changes'. See Chapter 7 for more on this.

There is no getting away from the fact that using this skill depends on you feeling confident about your authority, which we've already looked at in Chapter 2. Each skill requires you to use slightly more of your *personal* authority and none more so than constructive assertion. Your use of translation is still essential here, otherwise you won't be able to refer to implications that you know your colleague/s care about. Here, you are not using this understanding to convince someone logically but to require that they take a particular course of action. Maybe you won't need to use constructive assertion, particularly with a longer term influencing intention. However, it may be just the approach you need for a particular incident and is a helpful last possibility when you have tried just about everything else.

- How do you rate yourself out of 10 on constructive assertion as a skill?
- How can you use this to benefit your current influencing agenda?

One thing to notice about all these skills is that they involve you *directly* influencing those you need to engage. This might not always be either possible or optimal so what then? That's when we need to think about your influencing strategies.

Influencing strategies

What do we mean by an influencing strategy? Well, just as all healthcare organisations have a vision and a supporting strategy to describe how they plan to achieve it, so you have an influencing aspiration and need a supporting plan. What are the steps and stages, the sequence of events, the significant conversations and presentations that you anticipate will achieve your aspiration? Most of us underprepare to achieve change through influence; why would we leave something so important to chance?

- Before we go any further, please spend a few minutes jotting down who you critically need to influence to achieve change.
- As you do this, distinguish those you already have a good relationship with in green and those you don't enjoy such a good relationship with (either because you don't see eye to eye or simply because you don't come into direct contact with them frequently) in red.
- With this distinction in mind, then consider what you need to do, who you need to speak to and in what order in order to successfully influence.

Through working with nurse leaders as they progressively influence, I have noticed that there are three common strategic misconceptions that inhibit success, so let's focus on these now.

The first is a diffidence about contacting a healthcare colleague when they are either much more senior or not in our day-to-day network. Now this is interesting as, if we think about the importance of courage, then surely an important service innovation that is not gaining traction merits what I'll describe as social boldness? Even if you don't know someone, why impoverish patient care because of a slight awkwardness?

Tracey, Deputy Director of Nursing in a CCG, was dissatisfied with her role and ambitious for service innovation. Looking for new opportunities for over a year and turned down for several successive roles, she was losing patience. Rather than continue knocking at closed doors, she decided instead to open a few. She made contact with several colleagues she had heard speak at conferences, asked for exploratory conversations with senior staff in NHS England and worked up her service improvement idea so that she could briefly – and enthusiastically – explain her thinking. She now has a new role in a national organisation, part of which involves implementing her idea.

'I realise, now, that new ideas need new roles creating for them. So, my challenge was less about finding the right role and more about creating it. Nobody was going to ask for something they were unaware of so my job became making sure they did.'

To support your boldness, or maybe to replace it if you decide that direct contact isn't going to work then there's the possibility of indirect influence. This is the second limiting assumption I come across – that if you can't affect a colleague's thinking directly then there's no way forward. Now this is where the idea of organisations as social networks can be very powerful. Cross and Parker (2004) challenge our notion of organisations as hierarchies, where we only influence in a linear way, and show, using their organisational 'heat map', how influence works more like a social movement, where we need to engage the 'tipping point' of 15–18% of colleagues (Gladwell, 2000) in order to create a natural momentum for change.

Maybe a trivial but topical example of this is the sudden explosion of the popularity of quinoa. Not so long ago, I couldn't pronounce it (keenwa not kwinoa) and didn't see it for sale anywhere; now everywhere I go I'm surrounded by quinoa salads – they have even appeared in the NHS Leadership Academy's lunches. Quinoa is over the tipping point!

The point here is to ask yourself who you know who will influence others for you in a cascade that will eventually reach those you most need to engage. Inherent in this way of thinking is the idea of the 'First Follower' who is socially connected and who will influence others for you. I cannot do justice to this idea in words without referring you to the lively YouTube clip called 'Leadership Lessons from a Dancing Guy'.

- Watch the YouTube clip 'Leadership Lessons from a Dancing Guy'.
- Now, ask yourself who are your First Followers?

Which links to the third limiting assumption: that we have to convince our greatest opponents in order to influence. As it turns out, this is an exhausting and pointless exercise. Edmonstone (2003) describes this very well in distinguishing those who have low/high energy and inclination to change their practice.

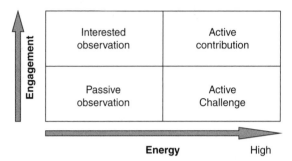

Figure 6.4 Inclination to change. Source: Reproduced with permission of John Edmonstone.

As you look at the model in Figure 6.4, please populate the categories with current colleagues and ask yourself where you invest most of your influencing attention and energies. If, as with many of us, it is with those in the bottom left-hand corner then please, from this moment on, change your strategy. By focusing your attention there, you are unwittingly saying 'these people's support matters more to me than everyone else's' and so disenfranchising others. Instead, the thinking behind this approach is that by investing in our cynics, spectators and players (for which, read First Followers), we are building engagement and the peer group will do the rest. It is much more likely that those who are 'victims' will be influenced by their peers' behaviour than by yours.

- How well developed is your influencing strategy?
- How far do you recognise the three limiting assumptions we have discussed?
- How can you use the ideas from this section to benefit your current influencing agenda?

The next and final section builds on this theme of rethinking our influencing assumptions by looking at how we can move beyond traditional influencing structures.

Influencing structures

- Think about how influencing for change normally happens in NHS organisations. What comes to mind?

What comes to my mind is the standard convention of a series of meetings and sea of papers comprising pages of words and meticulously framed verbal arguments. Clearly, there is a place for both but in this context, how can you offer something different to make your case not only compelling but also different, surprising even? This is where a little knowledge of the workings of our unconscious minds comes in useful. Back in the 1950s, there was frequent use of what was called 'subliminal advertising' – that is, advertising that is presented so briefly (for 0.003 seconds) that we are not consciously aware of it. Now banned in many countries, I am not suggesting that you revive it but that we can influence better by understanding some aspects of its effectiveness. So, alongside its rapidity, there were four important features: the fact that it stimulated interest through a question/suggestion, framed issues positively, was brief and mainly used images.

If you were to apply the first two of these characteristics to agenda building then you might, for example, be adding your item as a question rather than statement in order to arouse curiosity beforehand. Instead of 'Update on Patient Safety', you would offer an item on 'How can Mrs Hilman feel as safe as we want her to in our care?'. As well as generating interest, this framing also personalises the issue (the success of patient stories shows how much impact this has) and distributes responsibility amongst your colleagues.

The second two of these features could then transform most of our meetings. Rather than preparing another long paper, requiring hours of preparation to compose and read, why not offer a maximum of two sides of A4? You could use the popular SBAR (situation, background, assessment, recommendation) acronym as your framework.

'I was never sure how to write strong Committee papers,' says Gemma, Matron in a Foundation Trust. 'I always wrote too much and went into excessive detail to the point that I could see my colleagues' eyes glazing over!' She was delighted to come across the SBAR framework, used by many NHS organisations, during one of our Impact Group days, and now uses it as a template for all her reports. 'In a recent meeting, it took just 10 minutes to agree my recommendations using SBAR. Beforehand, discussions took so much longer and were often deferred. My written communications are much more influential now.'

Even more radically, you could use images or objects to influence. Both are extremely powerful approaches to making your suggestions felt and immediate as they involve our unconscious minds as well as more of our senses. Rather than describing the current and future state in words, you could show pictures of how things will be in the future compared with how things are currently, illustrated by the Hospital Pathways work I mentioned earlier in the chapter.

There may even be times when you can bring objects into the room with you to engage colleagues more fully.

Nancy is a Practice Nurse who wants to ensure that the very best use is made of all NHS resources. Having worked with Médicins Sans Frontières, she has seen great poverty and extreme suffering and speaks movingly about the daily miracles created by the prescription drugs we take for granted. Talking to her CCG Director of Nursing, she was horrified to find out how many prescriptions were regularly wasted and decided to do something rather unconventional about it, aiming to influence both her GP colleagues and members of the public. She decided to make the case tangibly.

Within the surgery, she uses an adapted and magnified blood pressure chart to indicate the changing levels of prescription waste to foster patient awareness. For CCG meetings, Nancy and her colleague leave illustrative empty drug boxes and bottles on the meeting table, accompanied by a simple question on a nameplate saying 'is this prescription really necessary?'.

I am aware that this section may contain some of the most unusual ideas of the chapter – which may signify its importance. Your influencing ambition deserves every idea you can muster so, as a final exercise, ask yourself:

• How can I use the ideas from this section to benefit my current influencing agenda?

At the outset of this chapter, I asked you to consider two questions: who do you want to influence about what and what gives you the right to do so? I hope that this chapter will have helped you to address the third and most challenging question, which is how you will successfully influence to improve patient care through your leadership.

References

Cialdini, R. (2007) *Influencing: the psychology of persuasion*. New York: HarperCollins.

Dent, F. and Brent, M. (2010) *The Leader's Guide to Influence: how to use soft skills to get hard results*. Harlow: FT/Prentice Hall.

Cross, R. and Parker, A. (2004) *The Hidden Power of Social Networks: understanding how things really get done in organisations*. Berkeley, CA: Harvard Business School Press.

Dickson, A. (1982) *A Woman In Your Own Right: assertiveness and you*. London: Quartet.

Edmonstone, J. (2003) Learning and development in action learning: the energy investment model. *Industrial and Commercial Training*, 35(1), 26–28.

Fisher, R. and Ury, W. (2012) *Getting to Yes*. Sydney, Australia: Random House.

Gallo, C. (2014) *Talk Like TED*. New York: St Martin's Press.

Gladwell, M. (2000) *The Tipping Point*. New York: Little, Brown.

Heron, J. (2001) *Helping the Client*. London: Sage.

Mehrabian, A. (1971) *Silent Messages*. Belmont, CA: Wadsworth.

Strozzi-Heckler, R. (2014) *The Art of Somatic Coaching: embodying skilful action, wisdom and compassion*. Berkeley, CA: North Atlantic Books.

Chapter 7 **Courageous conversations**

Jamie Ripman and Philippa Williams

'*Very great change, comes from very small conversations, held amongst people that care.*' (Margaret Wheatley, 2002)

'*A problem only exists in the absence of the right conversation.*' (attributed to Werner Erhard)

'*The conversation is the relationship.*' (Susan Scott, 2002)

These wise words reflect something that we suspect few would argue with: the depth of our relationships and the effectiveness of our leadership are dependent on the quality of the conversations we have. Our relationships with others are built piece by piece through the interactions we have, which of course include many different conversations. These can be corridor conversations, chats over coffee, meetings, appraisals, hand-overs, bed planning and so on. They will be conversations with patients, with other healthcare professionals, with relatives, with your line manager, with members of the admin team and many more. It sounds obvious, perhaps because it's the water we swim in and perhaps because many of those interactions are focused on the task, on getting the job done. So we don't stop to think deeply about them because there is no time or apparent need. Yet all these interactions count. As Ken Blanchard (2002) wrote: 'While no single conversation is guaranteed to change the trajectory of a career, a business, a marriage, or a life, any single conversation can'. And sometimes it might be a series of conversations that makes the difference.

'*I used to find it difficult going to the wards. Everyone suddenly went on red alert and put their gloves on. "What's wrong? What have we done?" I hated it because I just want to be liked! But I kept chipping away – just*

How to be a Nurse or Midwife Leader, First Edition.
Edited by David Ashton, Jamie Ripman and Philippa Williams.
© 2017 John Wiley & Sons, Ltd. Published 2017 by John Wiley & Sons, Ltd.

dropped in for 10 minutes and said "Anything I can help you with? Any questions?". Then I got back from maternity leave and was greeted with open arms – they said "Nobody comes down to see us any more".'
(Infection Control Lead Nurse)

Inevitably we find some people easy to deal with and some more difficult and the conversations we have will reflect that, as they are likely to reflect how busy we are, how we are currently feeling and what our current priorities are.

The title of this chapter is 'courageous conversations'; this implies that some conversations need courage, which in turn implies that these conversations will be the ones we perceive as 'difficult'. This might be breaking bad news to a patient or relative and it might also be challenging some behaviour in a colleague, or making a request of your line manager, or managing the performance of one of your team. And when faced with 'difficult' issues, many of us experience a tension; on the one hand, saying too little and avoiding the issue, on the other hand, saying too much, upsetting people and jeapordising a working relationship.

The authors of this chapter, Jamie and Philippa, started working within the NHS many years ago. A story, told by the late Professor Aidan Halligan, has stuck with us from the early days as an example of leadership in practice. The story concerns a ward round on a care of the elderly ward, led by a professor. There were about 12 people on the ward round, including the youngest member, a newly qualified nurse. They stopped at the bed of an 84-year-old man who was confused and probably suffering from dementia. Unfortunately, the young doctor who was speaking about him also became confused. The professor became impatient and eventually turned to the group, saying 'I'm fed up dealing with these stupid people'. Everyone suddenly became extremely interested in their shoes, nobody said anything, and the professor walked away in irritation. But after the ward round, the young nurse (who incidentally was an ex-estate agent who had retrained at the age of 24) found a moment to catch him and said: 'Nobody speaks to patients like that on my ward'. I'm sure you will agree that this was an act of courage on the part of this nurse. When Aidan told the story, he stopped there and asked the audience, 'What do you think happened next? Did this nurse have a job within the next six months?'. He also asked, 'How do you think the professor responded?'. The answer was yes, she did keep her job – and she became a sister on that ward soon after. And the professor apologised to her at the time: he said 'I'm really sorry, I had a row with the kids this morning. Let's go back and apologise to the patient together'. He was not a bad man, he had just reacted badly under stress.

'Our lives begin to end the day we become silent about the things that matter most.' (attributed to Martin Luther King)

Aidan's story, which is a true one, is a great example of a courageous conversation in practice, which had far more positive outcomes than the young nurse might have expected when she chose to speak out. Let's explore another example in a bit more depth.

Imagine it's the beginning of the day on a busy specialist stroke ward. Jackie Hanson is a ward sister who has put aside some time to do some administration. She is continually interrupted by phone calls so is feeling a little fraught and then one of the junior nurses, Mirembe, arrives in tears. She tells Jackie that the consultant (Simon Garner, a relatively new appointment who has replaced Tanvi, a very well-liked and respected consultant) has shouted at her. He was running late in his ward round, she tried to raise the issue of protected mealtimes with him and he reacted angrily. She claims that it's not the first time that he has done so. 'He shows me zero respect,' she says. She also tells Jackie that she's thinking of asking for a transfer to a different ward as a result of Simon's behaviour. This is also not the first time that Jackie has heard similar stories and, indeed, has experienced Simon being a bit brusque herself. She knows she has to say something to him. She manages to catch him in the corridor and asks him to drop in to see her, which he does (begrudgingly, she feels) towards the end of the day. The resulting conversation goes a bit like this.

Simon: What did you want to talk about? I'm in a bit of a rush.

Jackie: Please sit down, Simon.

Simon: I'd rather stand, if it's all the same to you.

Jackie: I wanted to talk to you about your ward round earlier. I had one of my staff nurses in who was quite upset.

Simon: Who? Why was she upset?

Jackie: It was Mirembe. She said that you had a go at her.

Simon: I don't think so …

Jackie: Well, like I say, she was very upset … she said you were very dismissive of her opinion and she says you snapped at her.

Simon: Jackie – I'm sorry if she was upset but I have a job to get on with. And anyway, I didn't snap at her … from memory, she was trying to make some point about mealtimes, I felt it was irrelevant and so I moved on to the next patient.

Jackie: Well, she says you snapped – and anyway, how do you know it was irrelevant if you didn't speak to her about it? And it's not just that, I've seen you be dismissive with other people as well …

Simon: When?

Jackie: Look, my point is you are very different to Tanvi in your style. Tanvi was very popular with the nursing staff.

Simon: And I'm not? I didn't know it was a popularity contest.

We'll leave them there at this point and come back to them. In the meantime, consider the following questions.

- What are you thinking and feeling about how Jackie handled this conversation?
- What are you thinking and feeling about Simon?
- How do you think Jackie was feeling?
- How do you think Simon was feeling?
- What might his intention have been?
- How would you have handled this conversation?

You'll notice that there are a lot of questions about feeling. What's your response to that? For example, are you thinking 'it doesn't matter how they're feeling, they should behave professionally', or 'they should be able to manage their feelings', or 'they're both obviously feeling bad and need to acknowledge that to themselves and the other person'? Or none of the above and something completely different!

The point here, of course, is that, whether we like it or not, feelings and emotions are part of our everyday interactions and drive our behaviour – sometimes in more ways than we wish to admit. In nursing, or indeed any kind of medical, social or clinical care, the 'emotional labour' (referred to in Chapter 1) that is needed can be overwhelming at times. The research that has been done on emotional intelligence (for example, by Daniel Goleman, 1996) explores how the most effective leaders are able to harness their emotional intelligence through self-awareness, self-management and empathy with others.

Our focus in this chapter is exploring how we can create the best conditions to enable us to have the conversations about the things that matter most. We will explore practical approaches to managing conflict and diversity of opinion, working with emotion, creating learning conversations and having effective conversations about performance. We will look at how we can plan and prepare for difficult conversations as well as seizing time 'in the moment' when appropriate.

We have structured the remainder of the chapter into three sections: Managing Conflict, Compromising and Collaboration, and Effective Conversations about Performance.

Section 1: How to manage conflict

Before we continue with this section, we invite you to undertake a short exercise.

1 Write down your definition of conflict.
2 Write down a few words to describe how you feel when you experience conflict.
3 Describe your preferred approaches to dealing with conflict by completing this sentence: 'Whenever I experience conflict I tend to...'

In our work with individuals and groups on managing conflict, we have had a wide variety of responses to these questions. In terms of a definition, the spectrum can range from 'being at war' to 'having a mild disagreement'. The feelings generated when experiencing conflict can range from feeling nervous, sick and stressed to feeling energised, excited and confident. Not surprisingly, therefore, personal preferences for how to approach conflict also vary significantly.

A quick search of online dictionary definitions of conflict reveals the following.

> 'A serious disagreement or argument, typically a protracted one' (www. oxforddictionaries.com) 'an active disagreement between people with opposing opinions or principles' and 'fighting between two or more groups of people or countries' (http://dictionary.cambridge.org)

Clearly, the word 'conflict' means different things to different people and will have different significance depending on your context. Of course, we are trying to define conflict in the context of nursing and midwifery leadership and, for us, there are some helpful reference points that have guided our thinking and our approach to working with nurses and midwives on handling conflict. Two such bodies of research are those done by Dr Elias H. Porter who developed his Relationship Awareness Theory® (Porter, 1996) which has since been developed into the Strength Deployment Inventory® (SDI®) (Porter, 2005), and the work done by Drs Kenneth Thomas and Ralph Kilmann which has resulted in the development of the Thomas–Kilmann Conflict Mode Instrument (TKI) (Thomas and Kilmann, 1974).

The SDI is a helpful diagnostic tool that we have used with individuals and groups that can help to create greater awareness about how we deploy our personal strengths at times when things are going well for us and also when we are in conflict or opposition with others. There are plenty of published resources available in print and online (www.personalstrengths.uk).

One helpful distinction that we have come across through this research is that between what they call 'warranted' and 'unwarranted' conflict.
- *Warranted conflict* – occurs when the people involved do not agree on the desired outcome.
- *Unwarranted conflict* – occurs when there is agreement as to the goal, but disagreement about the approach to accomplishing the goal.

Other chapters of this book (particularly Chapters 4 and 6) also deal with how we organise and energise others around a common purpose and goal and, in this chapter, we are also going to explore the challenges arising from unwarranted conflict, where a common purpose and the outcomes have been broadly agreed but the conflict arises due to differing styles, approaches, personalities and preferences.

In our experience, the theory and practical application of the TKI is a very helpful guide to get us started. So, our aim here is to give a brief introduction to the TKI and to encourage you to do further research and personal diagnosis. Again, there are plenty of published resources available (www.kilmanndiagnostics.com).

Let's start with their definition of conflict, which is 'Any situation in which the concerns of two people appear to be incompatible'. For us, this is a helpful definition as it refers to 'concerns' and to 'apparent' incompatibility. What concerns somebody is not always evident from their behaviours, as can be seen in our imagined scenario between Jackie and Simon. Jackie may have a hunch about her differing and apparently incompatible concerns with Simon but it feels like both parties are responding more to the strategies, language and behaviour of the other rather than investigating each other's underlying concerns.

How did you respond earlier to our questions about your thoughts and feelings about Simon? How would that affect your behaviours should you need to resolve any differences with him? If Jackie is thinking and feeling that Simon is 'typically arrogant and disrespectful to nurses', we can imagine that her responses are partly governed by this belief about him. Thinking about the Thomas–Kilmann definition of conflict, we believe that if Jackie is going to help resolve the apparent conflict between them, she will need to become more interested in Simon's underlying concerns and be less affected by his behaviours, which may be caused by multiple factors, some of them unrelated to the issues that Jackie wants to address.

However, sitting down with Simon and exploring his underlying concerns is only one strategy available to Jackie. What else might she try? Again, we think the TKI offers us some helpful pointers. It invites us to explore our options for responding to conflict along two different dimensions.
- The extent to which we seek to satisfy our own concerns – *assertiveness*.
- The extent to which we attempt to satisfy the concerns of others – *co-operativeness*.

In Figure 7.1 we show those dimensions expressed graphically along with the five modes or styles of handling conflict associated with this framework.

So, there are five different options available to Jackie. What might they look like and when might they be appropriate? And that latter question is crucial. One of the discoveries we can make when we explore the TKI for ourselves is a greater awareness of our preferred styles of handling conflict. Once we've got a greater understanding of this, we can start to become more aware of whether we are using our preferred styles appropriately or not and whether we might make some conscious decisions to use a style that is more appropriate for the situation. It's generally the rule that we are more skilful at

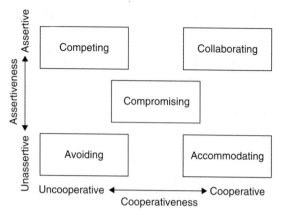

Figure 7.1 Thomas–Kilmann Conflict Mode Instrument. Source: Thomas, K.W. and Kilmann, R.H. (1974) *The Thomas–Kilmann Conflict Mode Instrument (TKI) Assessment.* Santa Clara, CA: Xicom, Inc. Reproduced with permission from the publisher, CPP, Inc. Copyright [1974]. All rights reserved. Further reproduction is prohibited without CPP's written consent. For more information, please visit www.cpp.com.

using our preferred styles (of anything) because we are more practised at them – even our bad habits! For the next part of this chapter, we want to explore what three of these five options (Avoiding, Accommodating and Competing) might look like, in practice, when executed with skill by Jackie. We're going to look at the strategies, behaviours and mindset required to be skilful at Compromising and Collaboration in the next section.

Avoiding
When to use
- When an issue is trivial or when other, more important issues are pressing.
- When you perceive no chance of satisfying your concerns.
- When the potential costs of confronting a conflict outweigh the benefits.
- To let people cool down.
- When gathering more information outweighs immediate action.
- When others can resolve conflict better.

How to execute with skill
To execute this style skilfully, it really helps to create a constructive mindset about your choice of this strategy. Be positive about your reason for using it – to yourself and to others.

In our scenario, Jackie may not have considered that it could be a helpful strategy to employ some appropriate 'avoiding'. Quite understandably, she has responded to a distressed member of her team and initiated some contact with Simon. She could have avoided doing this so quickly, recognising that her behaviours might still be affected by her negative feelings about his behaviour. On reflection, she might have considered avoiding the conversation for an hour or so until she felt calmer and had done some further planning for their first encounter after this incident.

Accommodating

When to use
- When you realise that your perception of the situation isn't helping.
- When the issue is much more important to the other person than to you.
- To build up credits for later use.
- When you feel outmatched and losing.
- When preserving harmony is important.
- To allow others to develop and learn from their mistakes.

How to execute with skill
Again, it's important to create a positive mindset about your use of this strategy. If 'backing down' or 'giving in' or 'admitting defeat' are the last things you would ever consider doing, then you'll need to create a different mindset about satisfying the concerns of others. In his research into the 'science of persuasion', Robert Cialdini (2001) identified 'reciprocity' as one of the deeply rooted human drives to which we can appeal when seeking to persuade others. It appears that humans are likely to reciprocate in kind, and if we offer an act of kindness or generosity to another person, we stand a better chance of getting something positive in return.

So, how might Jackie 'accommodate' with skill as part of her strategy of influencing Simon? Let's look at the issue of protected mealtimes that, in this scenario, led to the original incident between Simon and the junior nurse, Mirembe. Whilst holding firm to her belief of the importance of protected mealtimes, what if Jackie accommodated Simon's need to work at pace by offering him the following?
- He can have access to patients during mealtimes when he deems it essential.
- She will talk to her staff to explain the change of policy.
- She will monitor the impact of this on patients and get back to him if she feels it is having a negative impact on patient care.

If she was willing to offer this to Simon, our belief is that she could move on to the front foot with any eventual negotiation with him. She could proactively recognise and empathise with his need to work at pace, offer to help him out, and reiterate her passion not to compromise on patient care. According to Cialdini's research, she stands a good chance of Simon offering her something in kind in return.

THEORY INTO ACTION

Avoiding and Accommodating are both strategies where you are actively choosing not to satisfy your own concerns.

- In any of your own conflict situations, think of one example where you might consciously change your style and employ a constructive Avoiding or Accommodating style.
- Try it out.
- Reflect on your attempt at this change of style.
  - What were the benefits?
  - What were the negative consequences to you?
  - How might you refine your use of these styles to even greater effect?

Competing

When to use
- When quick decisive action is needed.
- On important issues where unpopular courses of action need implementing.
- On issues where you are determined to stick to your values and principles.
- To protect yourself against people who take advantage of non-competitive behaviour.

How to execute with skill

Competing is the high assertion and low co-operation style where you are aiming to satisfy your own concerns. There are many challenges to being skilfully assertive and we have provided a framework for having assertive conversations on our chapter on influence (see Chapter 6).

Another great thing about this assertive tool is that you can slide up and down the scale of assertion depending on how assertive you want to be. If we imagine assertion on a scale from 1 to 10, then up at the high end of that scale, where you have limited vested interest in the relationship, you can use words that are strong and direct. For example, if you are having problems of late delivery with a supplier of medical products to your department, you could be highly assertive about your request for change.

- We like your products and they are good value for money.
- We don't like the delays in delivery – sometimes as late as a month.
- So, we now need the deliveries to be made on time, every time.
- If you do, we'll continue to use you as our supplier.
- If not, we'll move to another supplier who offers a prompt delivery service.

In the case of Jackie, she definitely has an interest in developing her relationship with Simon and she will want to adapt her language whilst including the component parts to help her to be appropriately assertive. Here's our version of a short script she might write and memorise before starting the meeting with Simon.

- What I really appreciate are your plans for developing the stroke service and your passion and determination.
- What's concerning me is when this comes into conflict with established patterns on the ward and the impact on our nurses.
- What I want is a frank and honest conversation about the best way for us to work together.
- If you are willing to negotiate with me, I know we can help you achieve your goals.
- If we don't resolve this soon, my concern is that our nurses will disengage and it will be harder for you to realise your ambitions.

Jackie would then be ready to weave in these component parts during her conversation with Simon. She probably won't deliver this in one go but she has prepared the important elements and can include them at appropriate points in the meeting.

'I have found this assertion strategy enormously useful in a variety of situations and have shared it with all my ward/unit managers and nurse specialists, several of whom have been amazed by its effectiveness.

An example would be a staff nurse who I have had to speak to several times before about negative attitude to staffing and being very vocal in front of ward visitors about staff numbers on the ward. Previously conversations with her about behaviour were quite difficult and ended with neither party feeling happy with the outcome. Using the assertion format has gone something like this:

"I really appreciate your passion and I understand you feel strongly about patient safety and supporting your colleagues. However, it's not always effective to express your feelings to everyone on the ward or in front of patients. I would really like it if you speak to the ward manager about your concerns in a more private environment and we can try to address them. Would you like to join some of the work stream groups looking at safer staffing levels across the trust, maybe do some work with the acuity groups as I think your passion and insight into ward staffing issues would be really valuable?"

This person is now working on some of these work streams and has expressed their feeling that it was good to be listened to and feels that they have had some good input into the trust safer staffing strategy.' (Surgical Matron)

In Section 3 of this chapter, we will look at how to respond to the potential emotional reactions that can arise when we offer feedback to others. No matter how skilful you become at giving assertive feedback, you will also need to be ready for some very natural emotional responses to hearing an assertive request for change.

THEORY INTO ACTION

Think of a situation where it would be helpful for you to make an assertive request of someone. Use the guidelines above for how to structure an assertive conversation to prepare the component parts of your 'script'.

- Write down your assertive script.
- Practise the script out loud with congruent physical and vocal energy and refine if necessary.
- Learn the script sufficiently so that you can incorporate it easily into your conversation.
- Assess the pros and cons of having the conversation.
- If you are clear you want to go ahead, commit yourself fully to the style and be clear about your positive intention behind having the conversation.
- After having the conversation, reflect on what happened and how you can improve on what you achieved.

Section 2: How to compromise and collaborate

The two styles of handling conflict in the TKI that we haven't yet explored are Collaborating and Comprising. This is moving us into the 'win-win' territory of courageous conversations that we often aspire to occupy.

The decision between whether to collaborate or compromise will be different depending on the situation and the time and resourcea available. Here are some indicators.

Collaborating
When to use
- To find an integrative solution when the concerns of both parties are too important to be compromised.
- To merge insights from people with different perspectives on a problem.
- To gain commitment by incorporating others' concerns into a consensual decision.
- To work through hard feelings that have been interfering with an interpersonal relationship.
- When the objective is to learn.

Compromising
When to use
- When goals are moderately important but not worth the potential disruption of using more assertive modes.
- When two opponents with equal power are strongly committed to mutually exclusive goals.
- To achieve temporary settlements to complex issues.
- To arrive at an expedient solution under time pressure.
- As back-up mode when collaboration/competition fails.

How to execute with skill
Importantly, in our view, before we get to decisions about whether to compromise or collaborate, we feel it's essential to learn how to engage with others in a way that removes any potential blame, criticism or attack from the conversation. We explored the idea of empathic inquiry in the last chapter in the context of influencing others – let's see how this works if we add in a further intention of keeping our conversations free of blame and apply it to the conversation between Simon and Jackie.

We often witness conversations around differences which focus on attempts to prove that 'I am right' and that 'you are wrong' in the different positions taken over a particular issue. In our education, we are often schooled in having logical debates that will persuade others that our rationale is more powerful than another's.

An alternative strategy is to recognise that my position is only one version of reality, one 'perspective' on the situation, and that it is legitimate for you to have an alternative perspective.

> *'This is true AND this is true. Multiple realities are not competing. They just exist. You own a piece of the truth, and so do I. Let's figure out what to do.'* (Scott, 2002)

Informed by the wisdom gleaned by the research of Roger Fisher, William Ury and Bruce Patton (1992) and Susan Scott (2002), we have been experimenting with a framework for having blame-free, collaborative conversations that are proving to have some success. There are, of course, strong links here back to our chapter on influencing.

> *'I've been practising NOT jumping in with solutions and getting to know how others feel about the situation. I always found negative people difficult to deal with; people who cannot immediately grasp the advantages used to really annoy me. With practice, I have been able not only to see their points of view, but patiently accept starting from where they*

actually are. I have led a recent demanding pilot project in our CCG and spent a lot of time "holding hands" with anxious nurses. This time has paid dividends as 88% have completed the challenge, many to a very high standard, and are now, by their own admission, confident and prepared for the real thing.' (Nurse Practitioner and CCG Locality Nurse Member)

Let's build this framework using Jackie and Simon's conversation as an example. If we consider their respective opening 'positions' for this conversation, we could characterise their differences as follows.

Jackie: Protecting mealtimes is vital and you are a bad person for treating my staff like that. Tanvi would never have done that.

Simon: Protected mealtimes are irrelevant and your nurse wasn't being helpful to me. Comparing me with Tanvi is insulting.

In the scenario, we can see how both parties are sticking to these positions and having a 'yes, but ...' type of conversation in which they are trying to out-reason each other over the 'rightness' of their respective positions.

Step 1: Blame-free inquiry

Do you remember this quote from Chapter 3? 'Seek first to understand, then to be understood' (Covey, 1989). If Jackie is going to break this pattern, she could try exploring Simon's reality without laying blame. We shared this quote with you in Chapter 5: 'The person who can most accurately describe reality without laying blame will emerge as the leader' (Scott, 2002). To do this she needs to inquire into Simon's version of reality without judging his reality as right or wrong, good or bad. Her questions need to be genuinely exploratory and she will need to listen empathically to his responses.

> *'Most people do not listen with the intent to understand; they listen with the intent to reply. They're either speaking or preparing to speak. They're filtering everything through their own paradigms, reading their autobiography into other people's lives.'* (Covey, 1989)

Step 2: Summarise the reality of the other person – without laying blame

This is often a magical moment in a collaborative conversation. If your inquiry has been free of blame and you have listened empathically, you are now in a position to summarise back to your colleague 'the world according to them'. You are not agreeing or disagreeing with them; you are demonstrating that you have heard and understood their reality.

Here's how that might go for Jackie.

'So, Simon, what you're saying is that you're under a lot of pressure to develop the stroke service here and, consequently, you've got a huge amount on your plate. You are working at a furious pace and when Mirembe challenged you over protected mealtimes, you felt she was being unhelpful and it seemed reasonable to you to speak to her in that way.'

Sometimes you will discover that the other person's reality includes a perspective about you that will be difficult to hear and very different from your intentions. Try hard to resist the temptation to defend yourself at this stage and, instead, add this as part of your summary of the other person's perspective.

In Jackie's case she might say:

'And you're feeling frustrated with me for requesting some time to explore this when you're so busy.'

The great thing about developing the skills to make this sort of summary in courageous conversations is that you don't have to get it right first time. If you haven't accurately summarised your colleague's reality, they will correct any errors and you will often get some extra information into their perspective on things.

Assuming that Jackie has got to the moment in the conversation where she has accurately summarised Simon's reality, she will have arrived at what we sometimes refer to as the 'absolutely' moment, as that is often how the other person will respond at this point!

'Now what?' we hear you wonder! Well, often what is needed now is what you might call … an elegant transition!

Step 3: An elegant transition

This is a transition from blame-free inquiry about the reality of the other person to a blame-free disclosure of your version of reality. It's really important that this bit doesn't sound like 'That's great, now let me tell you why you're wrong!'. The language here needs to reflect your ultimate desire to build on the common ground between your realities, to acknowledge where your perspective is different and to offer your positive intention to find a collaborated solution (or compromise, if necessary).

In Jackie's case it could go something like this.

'Thanks Simon, that's very helpful to understand your perspective. Let me tell you how I see things. There's a lot of common ground between us and I do see some things differently so please hear me out while I explain my perspective.'

Step 4: Blame-free disclosure

> 'Your version of reality is as good as anybody's. As you describe reality from your perspective, do not lay blame.' (Scott, 2002)

During this step, you are disclosing your perspective using language that doesn't blame, criticise or attack your colleague. We will explore the skills required to give (and receive) feedback in the next section of this chapter so, for now, try this as an exercise. You don't have to have the conversations for real … yet!

THEORY INTO ACTION

- Go back to the scenario between Jackie and Simon at the start of this chapter and read the text a few times.
- When you feel you have understood Jackie's perspective, try to articulate it in a way that doesn't sound critical of Simon.
- How have you adjusted your language to enable Simon to hear your perspective without feeling the need to defend himself?
- Think of a situation that you are facing where your perspective is different from others. How will you articulate this in way that doesn't sound critical of others?
- Make a start. 'Let me tell you how I see things …'

Step 5: Share your desire to collaborate (or compromise)

Once you have each shared your perspectives on the situation, it is important to express your desire to build on the common ground you have uncovered and to work through the differences. We are not yet at the point of agreement or resolution of differences but we have avoided the tit-for-tat or 'yes but …' scenario where we started. To echo the sentiment from Susan Scott, you have described the reality of both parties, without laying blame, and you have emerged as the leader in this conversation. You are now well placed to lead the conversation that moves towards compromise (where each party gets some of their needs met) or full collaboration (where each party gets all their needs met).

Our recommendation for how you lead the next part of the conversation is to invite the other person to work with you to generate ideas for how to take things forward for mutual benefit. Let's finish this section by imaging how Jackie might lead Simon into the next part of the conversation.

Jackie: That's my take on things, Simon, and, as I said, it feels to me like we have a lot of shared views about the stroke service. We're both absolutely committed to make it the best we can and I appreciate there are a few differences between us in terms of how to do that. I'm really keen to develop our working relationship and to (either) find some compromises (or) collaborate with you. What are your thoughts?

Simon: I'd agree. It was helpful to hear your views but I'm not sure where we take things from here.

Jackie: Can we put aside a bit of time to explore that? I'd really like to work with you to generate some options for organising things a bit differently; I'd be happy to take a look at how you and the other consultants work with my ward team and me. Generate some different ideas and see if we can find some solutions that work for all of us. How does that sound?

Of course, we can't guarantee the extent to which Simon will engage with Jackie and she is still likely to need the range of influencing skills and strategies explored in Chapter 6.

What would be your approach at this point?

In our experience, this structure for having blame-free conversations has helped nurses and midwives to move courageously from the despair of wrestling with a challenging conflict situation into the possibility of negotiating a positive way forward. Here is one of the many examples that have been reported back to us.

'I have a member of staff who was being very distracted by issues away from work. She was making a lot of mistakes and causing other people a lot of extra work; showing a definite lack of interest at work and being very inconsiderate towards her colleagues. This was causing discomfort in the team.

I was able to confidently sit down with her and explain I had serious concerns. I was very honest and told her I felt she just did not want to be here, which is fine but unfair on the team when it affects work and the team dynamic. It prompted her to be honest about her issues and we were able to have a really open and honest conversation. She looked visibly relieved when we had talked, like a weight had been lifted. And I had a better understanding of why she was behaving as she was.

We made plans to help and support her. Ultimately this turned things around and she is back to her old self again, the team are happier and less stressed out too.' (Pulmonary Rehabilitation Clinical Lead, district care trust)

Section 3: How to have effective conversations about performance

I think people want to be magnificent.
It is the job of the leader
to bring out that magnificence in people
and to create an environment
where they feel safe and supported
and ready to do the best job possible
in accomplishing key goals.
This responsibility is a sacred trust
that should not be violated.
The opportunity to guide others
to their fullest potential is an honor
and one that should not be taken lightly.
As leaders, we hold the lives of others in our hands.
These hands need to be gentle and caring
And always available for support. (Blanchard, 2000)

Because the nurses and midwives we have worked with on this project have come from a range of grades and organisations, you won't be surprised to discover that the formal structures and processes in place for managing performance have varied significantly across their teams, organisations and trusts. You will have had your own experience of this both in terms of how your own performance is managed and also how you have managed others.

The way that some departments, teams and wards are organised has meant that we have met nurse and midwife leaders who have had as many as 40 staff to appraise. While we would recommend that no manager has more than 15 appraisals to do in a year, this chapter isn't aiming to tell you how to reorganise your staffing structures to help you keep on top of your appraisals.

What interests us are the regular interactions between leaders and the people for whom they are responsible. What can be done through regular conversations about performance to build the confidence, capability and, indeed, the magnificence of individuals and teams?

In this section we'd like to touch on a number of ideas that can help leaders to have effective conversations about performance. We'll cover:
• the cycle of performance conversations
• a structure for discussing and reviewing performance
• establishing clarity of the performance and standards required

- diagnosing the reasons for poor performance
- using appropriate management styles to develop performance
- guidelines for giving and receiving feedback
- dealing with the emotions involved.

The cycle of performance conversations

Your organisation will have its own formal cycle of appraisals and managing performance and it's important that you become familiar with this. A typical cycle goes something like the one shown in Figure 7.2.

As a leader in your system, you have an opportunity to model a positive attitude and culture towards managing the performance of others.

THEORY INTO ACTION

- What are the formal processes for appraisals and managing the performance of others in your trust?
- Where you are unsure, speak to a colleague in HR and ask them to get you up to speed.
- What is your current belief and attitude about the importance of having regular performance conversations?
- How is this reflected in your behaviours and strategies?
- What could you stop, start or continue to do to model a positive mindset and approach to managing the performance of others?

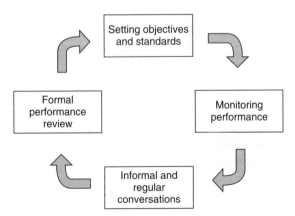

Figure 7.2 A typical performance management cycle.

As well as engaging in the formal processes that are organised by your trust, it is essential to have regular one-to-one catch-ups with your staff to explore how things are going for them and to discuss their performance. Ideally, these meetings should be once a week; they can be short and focused and an opportunity to consolidate or reinforce anything that has arisen in the last seven days.

It's important that performance issues are picked up as quickly as possible and you don't have to wait a week to appreciate someone for their high standards, positive attitude and putting in some extra effort. We have heard the argument that this is what is expected of nurses and midwives and thanking someone for doing a good job isn't appropriate. A more common belief is that there are not enough conversations of thanks, appreciation, success and good practice and, as a leader, you can have a significant impact on the culture of your team by regularly thanking and appreciating staff for their efforts. The other benefit of recognising and appreciating the efforts of others is that you will have credit in the bank when you need to address an issue of poor performance. This also should be done as close to the incident as possible. You don't have to wait a week before having a quiet word with a colleague if you have observed them falling below the expected standards. We'll explore this more in the section below on giving feedback.

A structure for discussing and reviewing performance
The aim with this approach is to have regular and informal conversations about performance so that both manager and team member come to formal performance meetings with 'no surprises'. These meetings often include some paperwork from the trust, which gives guidelines as to the structure of these meetings. These meetings, therefore, need good preparation with both parties ideally exchanging written evidence to support their perspective on the individual's performance. The introduction from the manager should include some clarity about the nature and purpose of the meeting, which will be different from the regular, informal conversations that have been taking place. Once both parties are settled into the meeting, it is helpful if the manager begins by asking the team member for their perspective of their own performance. See Figure 7.3 for a potential structure for these types of meetings. With regular, informal meetings taking place, it is very likely that the formal meeting will progress along the top line of this structure and move quickly to the formation of an agreed action plan.

If the meeting is moving into the lower parts of this chart, you can employ the strategies we explored earlier with blame-free conversations. Get interested in why you and the team member have different views and perspectives on their performance. Acknowledge where you are in agreement and where

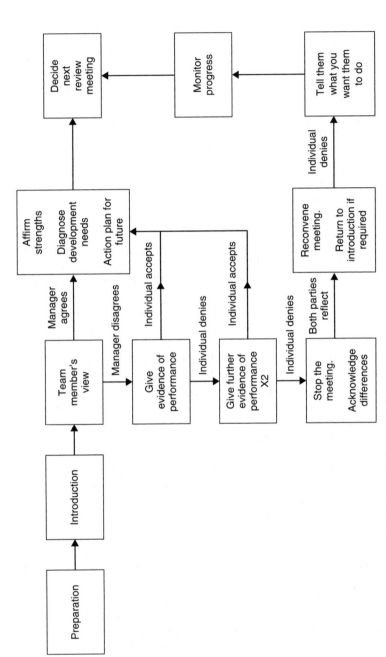

Figure 7.3 Discussing and reviewing an individual's performance.

there are differences and, if you feel the meeting is getting stuck around the differences of view, stop the meeting and ask to reconvene once you have both had a chance to reflect on things. This will sometimes allow you and the team member to break the emotional state of the meeting and the reconvened meeting can start with a fresh impetus.

The difference in this scenario is that if you can't resolve your differences with your team member, you now have positional authority to tell them what you want to happen and the benefits and consequences to them if they do or don't respond to your request. For us, this is a position of last resort and, to do this with skill, you can use the assertive structure we explored in Section 1. In a performance management context it can sound something like this.

I appreciate and respect that you are operating to the clinical standards expected of you. Where you are falling below the mark is when working under pressure you make remarks to other staff and to patients that they find distressful and rude. I want to be really clear about this – I expect you to put a complete stop to this from now on. If you do, I believe you can become a valued member of the team and your clinical skills will be even more appreciated. If you can't make this change you'll be falling below the standards expected of your role and we'll have to move towards a more formal process for managing your performance.

'The session on assertiveness was fabulous. I came back and showed it to my team; they all have it written in their diaries and use it all the time ... often on me!' (Pulmonary Rehabilitation Clinical Lead, district care trust)

Establishing clarity of the performance and standards required

In our experience, one of the challenges of managing the performance of others is helping individuals to get clarity about what is expected of them. The role of the manager here is to assess the performance of team members over time.

In the graph in Figure 7.4, we have plotted the performance of a newly qualified nurse, Jason, over time. Not surprisingly, Jason starts in the role below the standards expected of him; he develops to meet and then quickly exceed the expected standards and then his performance starts to drop and we end this period with his actual performance being well below what is expected. We'll come on to explore what might be causing this rise and fall of performance but the issue we want to look at first is how we get agreement about the expected standard. What are you doing to create a clear agreement with your staff about what is expected of them in their role?

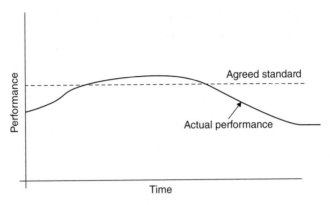

Figure 7.4 Establishing standards of performance.

Of course, there are a number of clear performance indicators and reference points that give guidelines as to what is expected. Here are a few.

- Job description
- Personal specification
- Trust values
- 6Cs
- The NMC Code

Your trust may have other indicators and there's often a lot to get your head around. It really helps to become familiar with these standards as they will assist you to identify quickly how an individual's performance relates to the standards. We're not suggesting an exhausting trawl through this literature with your staff but reminding individuals of these performance indicators can be helpful. An initial discussion that makes it clear that, as part of your role, you need to support them and hold them to account to meet these standards can allow you to return to these if you feel the standards are not being met.

This was brought to life for us recently when we worked with a trust on their Preceptorship programme. Providing the newly qualified staff (preceptees) with informative induction sessions and documents, a six-month probation period, ongoing support from a line manager, and up to a year of support from a nominated preceptor gave the newly qualified staff a clear understanding of what was excepted of them as they made the daunting move from being a student to a qualified nurse. Preceptors and line managers were encouraged to have regular conversations with preceptees about where they were exceeding, meeting and falling below the standards that were expected of them at that trust.

Diagnosing the reasons for poor performance

Let's return to our graph of Jason's performance over time (see Figure 7.4). We might reasonably expect that the lower than expected performance at the start is due to him getting up to speed with the requirements of the new role. As indicated, good induction and some clear direction at the start will enable Jason to meet and then, in his case, exceed expectations.

In a moment we'll come on to explore what might be causing the drop-off in Jason's performance but our questions for now are:

• How are you helping to induct new colleagues into their role?
• What more could you do?
• What are you doing to appreciate, support and encourage those members of your team who are doing more than is expected of them?
• What else could you do?
• What's the risk to you and them if you do nothing?

So, there's our first potential answer to the question about what might be causing the drop in Jason's performance. Without thanks, appreciation and further opportunities to develop and grow, he might have become disillusioned and lost interest.

We can only speculate about this and any other reasons why Jason's performance has fallen below the standard expected so let's do a more useful exercise.

• Think of somebody in your team who is not performing to the standard expected of them.
• Write down some specific examples of what they are doing and your explanation of why that is below the expected standard.
• Write down anything you know and any assumptions you have about why they are not meeting the standards.
• Looking at your list, try to divide your reasons into two different categories.
  • The first category is about ability: where does this person lack skills, competence or knowledge?
  • The second category is about will or attitude: where does this person lack motivation, confidence, commitment or the right attitude?

This diagnostic exercise can help you to identify the best style of leadership to use for developing your colleague. One way of thinking about the factors contributing to performance is look at the dimensions of 'willingness' and 'ability'. Ken Blanchard, who provided the quote at the start of this section, explores this to great effect using his Situational Leadership® model (Blanchard, 2001) and we encourage you to discover more through investigating this body of work (www.kenblanchard.com). Like many of the other models to which we refer in this book, there are tools available to help you to diagnose your preferred styles and reflect on whether you are using the best styles for the situation you are in.

Using appropriate leadership styles to develop performance

Taking some time to assess your staff's varying levels of motivation and skill, or willingness and ability (see Situational Leadership® above), can help you to make deliberate and appropriate changes in your leadership style to develop the performance of your staff.

The behaviours required for each of the styles are broadly as follows.

1 For staff who are motivated, keen and willing but lack skills and ability, take time to show them how to do things. Use a **Directing** style of leadership that can include the following behaviours:
   • Showing and telling how
   • Teaching and instructing
   • Checking / monitoring
   • Giving feedback.

2 For staff who are low in confidence or motivation and who also lack skills and ability, try a more **Coaching** style of leadership. This can include the following behaviours:
   • Exploring/asking
   • Redirecting
   • Praising
   • Encouraging.

3 For staff who have the skills and ability to do their job but lack confidence, motivation or the right attitude, you won't need to give them much direction. They have the skills already but need a more **Supporting** style of leadership to encourage and facilitate their development. This can include the following behaviours:
   • Asking/listening
   • Facilitating self-reliant problem solving
   • Encouraging feedback
   • Collaborating.

4 For staff who are motivated and willing and have the appropriate skills and ability, you need to find opportunities for them to spread their wings. This **Delegating** style of leadership can include the following behaviours:
   • Allowing /trusting
   • Empowering
   • Affirming
   • Challenging.

Review the work you did in the previous exercise.
- In which category of this model have you put the team member from the previous exercise?
- Which leadership style are you currently using to develop that individual?
- What could you stop, start or continue doing to help that individual develop further?

Guidelines for giving and receiving feedback
Giving feedback
Skilfully sharing your perspective about a situation or about the impact of the behaviour of another person is an important aspect of any leader's repertoire. Done well, it can be a powerful tool for influence and change. Done badly, it can be ignored and potentially harmful. Here are a few suggestions for how to keep refining your ability to give constructive feedback.

1 Always give feedback with a positive intention to help the other person.
- Resist the temptation to offer feedback when you feel the need to get something off your chest or because it will make you feel better.
- Phrase and time your feedback to give maximum benefit to the person receiving feedback.

> *Example: 'I want to share my perceptions of this with you because they seem to be different from how you are seeing things'.*

2 Focus on their behaviour, not their character.
- Try to describe the behaviour you have observed as objectively as possible and resist words or phrases that refer to any inferences you have made or to any judgements of character or personality.

> *Example: 'I've noticed you raising your volume and saying "as a junior nurse you need to understand …" on three occasions when you spoke to Mirembe' as opposed to 'You are very aggressive and patronising when you speak to Mirembe'.*

3 Distinguish between intention and impact.
- What you are giving feedback on are your perceptions of the other person's behaviours. As we discussed in Chapter 2, this is the 'impact' on you of what they are doing.
- It can help to understand or imagine what is the positive intention for the other person in behaving in this way. Think of your own behaviours and what motivates them. How often are you driven by an intention to cause upset or to do harm to others? For most people, it's the same. For Simon, what might be his positive intention for 'snapping' at

Mirembe? He is probably trying to deal with the challenge from Mirembe as quickly and efficiently as he can so that he can get on with his objective of seeing his patient. He may also not yet have learnt to do this with skill.

> Example: 'I appreciate you had an urgent need to see your patient. By responding in the way you did it came across that you didn't respect an important member of my team who was also trying to do her best for the patient'.

4 Take a positive approach to the other person's 'weaknesses'.
- Sometimes our weaknesses are our strengths that we overdo or misapply. Where this is the case, it can be helpful to acknowledge this.

> Example: 'I can see how determined and passionate you are to improve the service. I've noticed that sometimes that strong determination makes it difficult for you to respond to people who are offering a different perspective without sounding defensive'.

5 Don't overload.
- As we will explore in the next section, people take time to adjust to difficult messages.
- Plan the timing and amount of feedback to create maximum benefit to the recipient.
6 Get the other person to provide solutions where possible.
- Invite the other person to work out how they can close the gap between their positive intentions and any negative impact that is causing.

> Example: 'So how can you change what you're doing so that you keep your determination and passion and engage more with others who have a different perspective to add?'.

Receiving feedback

In the next part of this section, we offer some ideas for how to respond to others who might react emotionally to being given some feedback. It is a perfectly natural reaction and it can happen to all of us.

When it is your turn to be on the receiving end of feedback, be aware that your emotions might follow a similar journey to the one we will describe in the next section. So, when you are being given feedback try to:
- keep listening
- avoid jumping in with reasons and excuses
- ask questions to seek clarity on anything that isn't clear or for more detail if the feedback is too general

- give yourself some time to reflect on the feedback and absorb the messages
- add the feedback to other data you have on the situation
- create a constructive plan for how you are going to respond to the feedback.

Dealing with the emotions involved

Through your clinical work, you may be familiar with the work of Elisabeth Kübler-Ross, the Swiss-American psychiatrist who did pioneering work into the emotional reactions to death and dying, described in her book *On Death and Dying* (1969). In this book, Kübler-Ross explores the stages of grief and, in our experience, there are some similarities between this and the emotional reactions experienced by many people in response to hearing bad news of varying forms. For example, we've seen and experienced versions of this when observing people responding to assertive requests to change and other developmental feedback.

Of course, not everybody follows the pattern shown in Figure 7.5 precisely, but in preparing to give challenging feedback, it's also worth thinking about how you are going to respond should you encounter a reaction that includes elements of this emotional journey.

Sometimes it can be very challenging to be with someone who is experiencing these emotions and it's easy to make negative judgements of people when they subject us to their denial, blame or anger. This research and our experience show us that these are not bad people doing shocking things. These are typical people doing typical things and here are some ideas for how

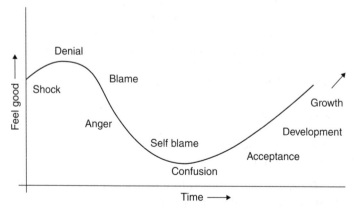

Figure 7.5 The Change Curve – people take time to adjust to difficult messages.

to care for yourself and the other person when they are in the grip of these emotions. To support someone through:

Shock: Empathise. The old adage is 'tough on the issue, not on the person'.

Denial: Repeat the message. Make sure the other person has clearly understood the feedback you have given. In the early stages of denial, it can be very tempting to rescue the other person and soften the message. This is very understandable and not helpful. The bad news for you is that by sticking to your guns, the situation is potentially about to get worse because once the message sinks in for your colleague, you are likely to experience an emotional journey from them that might include blame, anger, self-blame, etc.

Blame: Sometimes they will say it's the organisation's fault, sometimes it's the fault of other team members and sometimes it will be you who is being blamed. For example, 'Why didn't you tell me this earlier?'. Try not to take this personally and don't be inclined to defend yourself at this point. Encourage your colleague to tell you more.

Anger: Again, this can be directed at many targets. Your colleague will be speaking from a very emotional place (heart-felt) so try not to respond with reason or logic (head-space). Say as little as possible and listen hard. If anything, ask them to tell you more about what they are saying. Like a boiling cauldron, your colleague needs to vent their emotions and if you give them the time and space to do that, you can help them let off steam. Reasoning with them is like pushing down the lid on the boiling cauldron and they will retain their heat for longer. And remember, you can offer your colleague some time to think things through. Not everything has to be achieved in one meeting and giving them (and you) a break can enable you both to reconvene with a different energy.

Self-blame: Empathise and remain curious. How do they feel they have played a part in this?

Confusion: Listen and empathise.

Acceptance: Appreciate and encourage.

Development: Offer support.

Growth: Appreciate.

'I made a decision on working patterns because I wanted to increase the presence of the senior nurses on the shop floor during key working hours. The Matrons and Heads of Nursing wanted to work fewer days but

longer hours whereas I needed more senior people around during the day when some of the difficult things were being tackled like resolving bed-flow problems, seeing patients and talking to relatives. It was much better for patient care.

It was very challenging because I was breaking the set patterns of people's working lives and they reacted emotionally to this. There were tears, they wrote me an angry letter and they worked to rule for a while.

What I really valued through understanding the Change Curve was feeling reassured that I wasn't doing something badly; this was a normal response to the changes I had asked of them. I stayed calm, listened and empathised with their feelings, compromised on a few issues and, eventually, the angry reactions stopped as they accepted the changes.' (Divisional Director of Nursing)

We've been told many examples of nurses and midwives who have tried to address challenging performance issues with colleagues and found themselves on the receiving end of 'bullying' accusations. When someone is given a clear message about their poor performance and heard it for the first time, we think the Kübler-Ross research can help us to understand the range of emotions that this will provoke. It's tough on them and it can be tough on you too so we encourage you to be vigilant and honest with yourself about how you treat others when you are addressing issues of underperformance. In the heat of the moment, ensure that you are being assertive and not aggressive. It's your job to address issues of performance in your team and how you go about it is critical. We hope this chapter has provided some ideas, frameworks, tools and techniques that can help leaders to manage conflict and poor performance with skill and to prepare for courageous conversations. And here's a note of warning attributed to a nineteenth-century German Field Marshall, Helmuth von Moltke the Elder, that encourages us to keep learning from our experiences and to keep on our toes at all times:

'*No battle plan survives first contact with the enemy.*'

Even more courage required ...

Before we leave this chapter on courageous conversations, we'd like to return to the scenario between Simon and Jackie at the start of the chapter. The issues to which we haven't yet paid attention are the potential issues of power, equality and diversity arising from the gender, race and social background of the characters involved. Here are a few questions we'd like you to consider.

- When you read about the interaction between Simon and Mirembe, what did you envisage?
- Did issues of race, privilege, power and gender come to mind?
  - If so, why?
  - If not, why not?
- How have you reacted to us drawing your attention to this?
- How did you react earlier when we didn't draw your attention to this?

What we know is that issues of power, equality and diversity play into the dynamics of our relationships in the workplace. They are often difficult subjects to raise with others and to admit to ourselves. We will explore this topic further later in the book and it feels important to recognise that within your repertoire of courageous conversations, you will probably need to find ways of starting conversations that help to pay attention to this. As we finish this chapter, how about this as a courageous starter for Jackie?

'Simon, I've been speaking with Mirembe about helping her to become more influential on the ward. She's been very open with me about some cultural issues that make it difficult for her to speak up with confidence and I've been working with her and other members of the team to talk about this and explore how we can enable a better balance of contributions. Put simply, I want all the staff on my ward to be treated fairly and equally and I've observed that isn't always the case. I'm not saying this was a relevant issue in this case but I am asking for your support on this issue. How does that sound?'

References

Blanchard, K. (2000) *Situational Leadership® II: The Article*. San Diego, CA: The Ken Blanchard Companies.

Blanchard, K. (2001) *Situational Leadership® II: The SLII® Model*. San Diego, CA: The Ken Blanchard Companies.

Blanchard, K. (2002) Foreword. In: Scott, S. *Fierce Conversations: achieving success in work and in life, one conversation at a time*. London: Piatkus Books.

Cialdini, R.B. (2001) Harnessing the science of persuasion. *Harvard Business Review*, October, 72–79.

Covey, S.R. (1989) *The 7 Habits of Highly Effective People: powerful lessons in personal change*. London: Simon & Schuster.

Fisher, R., Ury, W. and Patton, B. (1992) *Getting to Yes: negotiating an agreement without giving in*. London: Random House Business Books.

Goleman, D. (1996) *Emotional Intelligence: why it can matter more than IQ*. London: Bloomsbury Publishing.

Kübler-Ross, E. (1969) *On Death and Dying*. London: Simon & Schuster.

Porter, E.H. (1996) *Relationship Awareness Theory®: manual of administration and interpretation*, 9th edn. Carlsbad, CA: Personal Strengths Publishing.

Porter, E.H. (2005) *Strength Deployment Inventory®: Standard Edition. Manage conflict and improve relationships.* Carlsbad, CA: Personal Strengths Publishing.

Scott, S. (2002) *Fierce Conversations: achieving success in work and in life, one conversation at a time.* London: Piatkus Books.

Thomas, K.W. and Kilmann, R.H. (1974) *The Thomas–Kilmann Conflict Mode Instrument (TKI) Assessment.* Santa Clara, CA: Xicom,.

Wheatley, M.J. (2002) *Turning to One Another: simple conversations.* San Francisco, CA: Berrrett-Koehler Publishers.

Part 3

Leading collectively and collaboratively

Chapter 8 **Moving between the dance floor and the balcony (Heifetz and Linsky, 2002)**

Nicholas Bradbury with additional contributions from Nichola Jacob

'I could have danced all night,' sings Eliza Doolittle in the famous song from *My Fair Lady* and you can no doubt think of other 'dance the night away' songs. Dancing is engaging, bodily, active and fun. Well, not all nursing is fun but it is always practical. Dancing is a response to music. Nursing is a response to people. It is engaging, bodily and active. Why would a nurse want to move from the dance floor to the balcony? Why stop the action to become an onlooker?

There is a good reason. No, an essential reason. To be a nurse leader, it is crucial to learn the mindset appropriate to leadership. You need a suitable framework for thinking. You need the perspective from the balcony to help you make sense of the whirling, ever changing movements of the dancers on the floor. You need a way of seeing things that guides how you be a leader. And, as the leadership guru Kurt Lewin said, 'There's nothing so practical as a good theory'.

As we say in our introduction, there is a strong argument to suggest that nurses and midwives are in the forefront of leading the healthcare service. Both in terms of numbers and by the centrality and quality of what you know and what you do, it behoves you to lead the service. So you above all must be sure to learn the most up-to-date mindset that leaders need. This is particularly important in the early twenty-first century because until recently, leadership has been dominated by ideas stuck in a largely dysfunctional paradigm, best described as the 'mechanical' paradigm. A paradigm/mindset is a framework for understanding things (Stokes, 1995).

> Where do you spend most of your time, on the dance floor or on the balcony? How often do you switch between the two?

How to be a Nurse or Midwife Leader, First Edition.
Edited by David Ashton, Jamie Ripman and Philippa Williams.
© 2017 John Wiley & Sons, Ltd. Published 2017 by John Wiley & Sons, Ltd.

The mechanical mindset

The challenge with this leadership paradigm is that it tends to see people more as if they were machines than as people with beating hearts and lively minds. This way of thinking has slipped almost unnoticed into our language: 'My organisation is like …': what word came into your mind? For many people, it was probably a mechanical image. 'My organisation is like a well-oiled machine.' 'My organisation runs like clockwork.' 'The machinery of government.' 'Policy instruments' or 'policy levers.' These phrases are embedded. We suspect there are ministers who quietly believe it's just like that; when I 'pull a lever' in Whitehall, my policy will roll out effectively all over the country. Poor ministers! What a surprise they get when some months later their Permanent Secretary informs them that their policy had the opposite of its intended result (Chapman, 2002). A good example would be a policy intended to reduce illicit drug use: the idea was to promote health and reduce crime by increasing customs vigilance so there would be less drug availability. The result was the opposite: health worsened because criminals cut these now more expensive drugs with bad stuff and crime increased because, being more expensive, there were more thefts and violent attacks to fund the addiction.

We are only at the start of diagnosing the problems with the mechanical paradigm. So far, we have noticed it operates mostly below the radar as embedded assumptions hidden even in language. And we have spotted that an apparently rational and seemingly sensible policy can have unintended consequences that clash with its purpose. Please bear these two ideas in mind as we continue: the limits of rationality and the frequency and potency of unintended consequences.

The mechanical model assumes that a human organisation is like a machine. You can build and dismantle a machine by manipulating its component parts. If a cog goes rusty, you can take it out and replace it. In this way, the mechanic has complete control over the machine. Early pioneers of management theory thought this way of being in control could be applied very nicely to human organisations like hospitals. The people equate with the components and cogs of the machine. All managers have to do is to place people in a hierarchy and give them a function with a given set of tasks and … bingo … the managers will have control! People can be disciplined or removed like rusty cogs. Plans can be made with timetables and penalties.

Where have you experienced a mechanical approach that has worked? What was the leadership approach taken?

Where have you experienced a mechanical approach to problem solving that hasn't worked? Why not?

Unfortunately for this approach, human beings are not machines (Wheatley, 1999). The idea that work is for work and love is for home is too extreme. People always need to be valued as people as well as functionaries. We need dignity, connection, affirmation, recognition, meaning, humour, challenge and support. When the organisation effectively tells us to leave our humanity in the car park on the way in because it just needs us to do tasks, it pays a terrible price. It has locked up our spirit in a function. It has imprisoned our energy in the confinement of our tasks. What about our imagination, initiative, generosity, creativity, passion and capacity to think? In any case, it is a fantasy to believe people will do what they are told and only what they are told. In 'the Beer Game', a famous simulation of four different beer-making companies where each operative in each company is required to do *exactly* the same thing, how come, after a good many rounds, one company generally does brilliantly, one pretty well goes bankrupt and two are somewhere in the middle? When the exercise is analysed afterwards, it's always because of the same thing: people don't obey instructions – they think! They think they have a good idea (order more malt for economies of scale) but they can't see the unintended consequences (their firm is heavily penalised for storage costs). Or else, being human, after a few rounds they get a bit bored and try out a new approach just for the heck of it.

People make different assumptions. We all have our own way of making sense of the world. You only have to watch the news to see that. The causes of wars and conflicts are not just rational, are they? Social and cultural determinants, history, the allegiances, ideologies and aspirations we learned through our upbringing, different personality types and so many variables bear witness to the saying that we do not see the world as it is, we see it as we are. This is true to the point that you can be an expert on some subject but dismissed by your conversation partner. I remember being in the pub once explaining something I knew well to someone with no knowledge of it. But they said, 'Neeeer, I don't agree with that' as if that put an end to the matter. Somehow my knockdown evidence had been reframed as irrelevant. To them it was just 'wrong'. It didn't fit their worldview.

So you can rarely know 'the facts' if, as we suggest, you espouse multiple perspectives, because different perceptions and interpretations will nearly always offer a different way of seeing things. As explored in Chapter 2, even something as easy to understand as the Myers Briggs Type Indicator® (MBTI®), which sorts personalities into extrovert and introvert and between other fundamental dichotomies, shows how sometimes other people we work or live with seem to be on another planet. And yet when you have experienced the way the MBTI determines differences, you can see the validity of different interpretations of the world.

> Think about some of the people you work with. How do they see things differently from you?

So when leaders try to implement perfectly rational decisions, it mostly goes wrong. Rational decisions don't work out because in real life the relation between cause and effect is uncertain. It is not linear. Non-linearity is enhanced by what are called nested feedback loops that undermine rationality. What goes around comes around. The boomerang you threw comes back and hits you in the face. You gave an order you were supposed to have the power to do, but the response you got was stroppy and subtlely non-compliant. In the end, what you were trying to do got utterly sabotaged. So actually, managers cannot after all predict outcomes. A simple example would be the 'feedback loops' embedded in context. Let's say a government minister regularly gives Sunday lunch to some friends who work in the field of health. And let's say they all live in Tunbridge Wells. Over lunch, they all agree on some idea for improvement that they have found works well in Kent. Well, to the minister it's obvious. This should be his policy. He tries to implement it, with disastrous results. What worked in Tunbridge Wells turns out not to work at all in Salford or Middlesbrough. There are just too many variables.

Needed: a new mindset to understand complexity and wicked problems (Grint, 2010)

A rule of thumb is that a mechanical approach may work for 'tame' problems but it will not work for 'wicked' problems. Let us explain: examples of tame problems would be how to mend a car, how to choose a move in chess or how to spot an error in a complicated set of accounts. Even engineering the Channel Tunnel or sending a rocket to the moon can be seen as tame problems, in that once you have worked out all the technical problems, like drilling through rock or safely returning to Earth's atmosphere, you can overcome those obstacles again and again in the same way. So the mechanical paradigm is still needed. It is still useful. It gave us much of the kit used by nurses every day, not to mention the technology allowing us to fly abroad for a much needed break. The problem comes, and it is all too common, when the mechanical paradigm, with its mechanical mindset, is used when the problem is wicked, not tame.

Wicked problems are unlikely to have 'a solution'. They are not a type of problem that can be 'solved'. For example, what is the solution to climate change, crime, war in the Middle East or world hunger? There is no solution. What we are working towards is better outcomes and not worse outcomes. A good everyday example would be bringing up children. The 'problem' keeps changing. The questions they ask keep developing. What parents are trying to influence keeps changing. And this is a permanent process. It does not stop when the children leave primary school, it probably gets worse! Bringing up children has gone beyond being complicated, it is complex. Its problems are wicked.

The difference between the two can be understood by thinking about predicting what will happen if you throw a rock and predicting what will happen when you throw a live bird. If an issue involves human beings and goes beyond the merely technical, it is likely to be more of a wicked problem. Managers and policy makers often do not understand this. Hospital managers and politicians often formulate policies as if they could be implemented with the predictability of throwing a rock. But human beings are much more like live birds than rocks.

So the question becomes, what would it look like to respect this, and so to manage and lead people while recognising their freedom, all the possibilities of their being human, their initiative, passion and what they themselves really care about?

Write a list of some of the challenges/issues you face: put them into two separate columns; one for tame, the other for wicked. What might be the different leadership approaches you could take to work with these challenges?

A systems mindset

Having read this far, you can see more clearly how a mechanical mindset can often be detrimental to leadership and hence to optimal patient care. When people feel controlled, put into a box, unable to find their autonomy or use their initiative, it shuts down all their capacity to innovate, it undermines their morale and takes away any incentive to go the extra mile. Obedience to micro-management isn't any fun. Fulfilling work is work that matters to you, has meaning and purpose and leaves you feeling that you've made a difference.

So if the mechanical mindset does not work for leadership, what might be a better metaphor? We are looking for a model that helps us empower, engage, inspire and stimulate those around us, rather than cramp their style. Help can be found in the science that has emerged over the last century. Subatomic physics, chaos theory and all the science around complexity and emergence may seem a long way from helping us practically, helping leaders. But hang in there. Let's make some connections.

Mechanical thinking frames things in terms of cogs and fitting together component parts. The newer sciences frame things in terms of relationships.

Building on work by Einstein, two scientists, John Bell in the 1960s and Alan Aspect in the early 1980s, carried out experiments that suggest relationships are not just essential for human beings; they are essential for the existence of the universe (Gribbin, 1984). Relationships lie at the heart of all reality. Simply put, this experiment was a simulation in which two electrons were paired but then separated by a huge distance, the equivalent of many thousands of miles. Then, when the spin of one electron was reversed, at the same instant the spin of its paired electron reversed itself to stay in synch. The message is, 'don't mess with relationships because if you do, you're messing with the basic structure of how the universe is built!'. At the moment physicists still don't know *how* this relationships works. But they know it's the relationship that counts.

It's the relationships that count

Everything's connected to everything else. A random example: the limestone of the Peak District in Derbyshire was once covered with sea just south (yes south) of the equator and is made up of the remains of the tropical fish and sea life inhabiting those parts around 300 million years ago. In our very late arrival as the human species, everyone's connected to everyone else. Everything is interdependent. We are an interdependent set of molecules living in an interdependent ecosystem. Chaos theory, with its famous image of 'the butterfly effect', is a complementary understanding. It introduces the idea that a butterfly flapping its wings in California (or wherever you like) can influence the weather in the Atlantic (or wherever you like). We can already begin to see how far-reaching the implications of the systems approach might be. Or can we? Wait a minute. This can't be serious. It's policies and procedures, protocols and rules that keep patients safe, not relationships. Hmmm. Not entirely. Let's investigate some more.

Quantum physics offers us the idea that although we possess many remarkable potential qualities, many of them lie dormant. Even the genes responsible for our uniqueness are not entirely predetermined. They need to be 'sparked' into life, so to speak, by a relationship with the environment. The idea of the self-fulfilling prophecy is well researched and well known. For example, if a teacher consistently adopts the attitude that a particular person in their class will do well, guess what, that person tends to do well. Conversely, if a teacher, consciously or unconsciously, does not believe in a pupil's aptitude or ability, that pupil is at serious risk of badly underperforming. In the 1960s there was a social experiment in a primary school known as 'Blue Eyes, Brown Eyes'. It would not be allowed today because it was manipulative and unethical by current standards. However, it pointed up loud and clear that children will swiftly see things differently and behave differently if a person in authority directs them to do so. In the documentary, the teacher tells the children that those with blue eyes are to be treated better and take priority in certain respects according to a number of rules. The speed at which the class falls into line is shocking. Then the same teacher reverses the directive so that the blue eyes now become subservient. Again the children fall into line. This is a negative story but it alerts us to positive possibilities.

Imagine you go into work early on a Monday morning after a good weekend and you see your most difficult and needy subordinate, Fred, walking towards you down the corridor. What do you feel? Your heart sinks, maybe. You think something like 'Oh no! This is the last thing I need on a Monday. What a dreadful way to start the week. He will nab me with his whingeing for at least five minutes now'. OK, very understandable. But now imagine that you find in yourself the generosity to see Fred with the mindset of quantum physics. So you see him as a bundle of dormant possibility. You imagine him if all his potential were fulfilled. You think what he could be if someone were to fall in love with him or if his mother had loved him more or if he had found more control and pleasure in his life so far. You treat him warmly and positively and find yourself able to feel really pleased to see him. You find a genuine expectation inside yourself that he could change, could grow into a more rounded person. Well, one thing is for sure: go up to him with your 'oh no' attitude and you'll get the same old Fred you've always known. Try the new approach and you may not get an instant miracle but you'll feel better inside and it may indeed be the start of a miracle for Fred. He has a chance to start to grow into the person he could be with more self-confidence and less inner hurt. How you see people strongly affects what you get from them.

> Set yourself the task of using this approach regularly over the next three weeks. What difference do you notice in yourself and your thoughts about the person? What difference do you notice in the other?

Do electric or magnetic fields care about walls? No. Why ask? Because again, a mechanical mindset has influenced how we think about organisations, prompting us to think of them as immoveable structures, like heavy machines or stone buildings. The enormous Shell building, for example, just behind the London Eye on the south bank of the Thames, suggests that Shell's identity as a powerful organisation is defined in stone for ever. In other words, we have come to think that the organisational environment is fixed. We might imagine there is not much we can do to change it. In fact, the opposite is true. We are creating the organisational environment all the time. And as with electronic or magnetic fields, there is no empty space. But there are patterns to the way the vibes work. OK, so 'vibes' isn't a very scientific word, but it's true, isn't it!

You can go back to, say, a hospital canteen where you worked ten years ago and people are sitting at tables still complaining about the same sort of things in the same sort of way as they were the last time you were here. Note the implications of the fact that 'there is no empty space': this presents you with a continuous opportunity. You can fill the space with what you care about. Leaders need to broadcast their key messages with passion, like they really matter! When you do this, you are filling the space and creating the environment. So if the bad news is that the vibes can regress, as in that canteen, the better news is that they can be massively improved by you as a leader using your influence in every conversation you have.

Organisations are like fish tanks
If you waggle your finger in the top left corner of a fish tank, the fish patterns change and the flora wave about. If you waggle your finger in the opposite corner the same thing happens. As Margaret Wheatley (1999) wrote, 'Organisations are full of interpenetrating influences and invisible structures that connect'. The organisational vibes are created by everyone. This is why, as we explored in Chapter 7, every conversation you have matters so much. You can influence behaviour.

One of the great advantages of abandoning the perspective of hierarchy and adopting the 'fish tank' perspective is that it doesn't matter where you are in an organisation, you can still have a powerful influence. True, a CEO can send out thousands of emails at the touch of a button. But that CEO has absolutely no control over what will happen to them. Some staff may have them on autodelete! In one influential organisation we know, the long-standing receptionist in charge of the front desk had an influence on the organisation entirely disproportionate to his position on the pay scale. He was a man of presence, dignity and innate authority. You didn't get past the front desk without his say so. That was his job. Yet when he thought something needed to change, he put in a word here, sent out a signal there, and more often than not what he suggested came to pass. We will come back to this in the next section on organisational culture.

So now we have metaphors to help us understand the systems mindset from three branches of modern science: subatomic or quantum theory, chaos theory and field theory. The mechanical mindset zooms *in* to see component parts. The systems or 'new science' mindset zooms *out* to see how everything is related to everything else. This is true in ecology, in subatomic structures, in weather systems and in all non-linear adaptive systems including complex human systems, the kinds that give rise to wicked problems. The new mindset understands that the essential features of an entity lie in its interconnectedness, not its component parts.

Emergence

This mindset helps us ask the question 'Are you making the most of your relationship?' which takes us close to the notion of synergy: the idea that an energy, possibility or capacity is more than the sum of its parts. Breaking something down into component parts helps you see how a machine is built. Zooming out to see interconnectedness helps you see the extra value you can get by fully exploiting every possibility of all your relationships. There is a word in science for this: emergence. This is the idea that parts of a system can do things together that they could not do alone. A good illustration for emergence would be to imagine you go into a scrapyard and, as it happens, by coincidence, lying in a heap are two wheels, a chain, some pliable metal and some other bits and pieces. As you look at this heap of parts, you almost immediately think, 'With a bit of work someone could assemble a bicycle out of this lot'. Now imagine it is before 1869, the year of the penny farthing's invention. The possibility of making a bicycle by placing wheels, a chain, handle bars and a saddle into the configuration of a bicycle has existed for centuries, but no one has ever thought of it or, in other language, *the concept has not yet emerged*. It was always a potential possibility; this heap of parts had what are called 'emergent properties'. What needed to happen was for someone to zoom out to see that potential, to see what else the relationship between all the parts could do if, as it were, it were given the chance.

This is a bit like what we know to be the case when we work in a high-performing team where we can almost feel the synergy: everyone is seamlessly collaborating and it really does feel that the team's achievement is much more than the sum of its parts.

Think of a time when you worked as part of a high-performing team (inside or outside work): what was it like to be part of this? What did you notice about the behaviours and the nature of the relationships within the team? How could you use this experience/knowledge in the team you are currently working with?

What does all this theory teach us? What does it mean in practice for how to be a nurse or midwife leader? This is what we need to think about next.

The 'dos' and 'don'ts' of leadership behaviour

If we gather up the lessons we have learned, we could summarise them like this.
- Don't try to control or micro-manage your staff as if they were cogs in a machine. It won't work and the quality of response you get from them will be poor.
- Don't try to control or even understand all the variables that make up the ingredients of an issue involving human beings. The issue is likely to be a

wicked problem. The relationship between cause and effect will be very uncertain. Understand that the idea that you can manage by control is a fantasy, whether you are a government minister or a ward sister.

- Don't imagine, when you try to implement even your best idea, that there will be no unintended consequences. If your idea involves people, there will be. Look out for them.
- Don't see your staff and colleagues just from the perspective of their role, function or place in the hierarchy. See them as fully human beings with huge potential.
- Don't underestimate the power of your capacity to influence in every conversation you have. It's almost certainly more than you think.

The 'dos' are mostly the inverse of the 'don'ts'.

- Do see things from many points of view. Analyse your own perspective critically to see what has influenced it. Where has this enabled you to see something clearly? Much more important, where might this vantage point have blinkered you? When someone says something and you find yourself spontaneously thinking 'Oh, that's definitely wrong', stop. Think. Don't be like the person who said, 'Well, I *could* agree with you but then we'd both be wrong'! Instead turn your judgement into curiosity. What is leading this other person to think their view is right? What might it possibly express that you are missing? What might be an advantage in seeing the issue this way? One of the fundamental skills of leadership is to be able to turn spontaneous critical judgement into curiosity. This virtue is closely allied to your capacity to accept other people for who they are. And this of course gets us into deeper water. Because how much you can tolerate other people depends largely on your capacity to accept yourself. As we explored in Chapter 5, where you have unresolved issues or little neurotic irritabilities inside you that stem from lack of self-esteem, bruising from the past or a failure to receive sufficient unconditional love in the early stages of your life, then your capacity to accept others will be circumscribed. And we all share limitations here in some regard. Overcoming our neurotic foibles is the work of a lifetime. But it is a journey leaders have to make as expeditiously as possible because the success of your leadership depends in large part on how well you manage it and how much self-awareness and self-knowledge you learn on the way.

The development of you as a person and the development of the skills you need as a leader belong together (Goleman, 1996). There is no better example than in this instance of how well you can transform judgement into curiosity. The ability to see multiple perspectives is a non-negotiable must-have for a leader, not a nice-to-have. So is the skill of weighing up a situation having examined all perspectives.

A good illustration for seeing how important this skill is would be to think of a hospital ward on a day when different demands and needs were competing furiously. A skilful nurse leader would be able to bring to bear not just their own subjective, sometimes unconscious, default priorities but an accurate assessment of the many perspectives from many starting points: safety, the characters of the staff on duty, clinical priority, patients' family issues, pressure from medics, corporate priorities, governance issues, management pressures, economics, best care for each patient … the list could of course be longer. Creating the best balance of response to these competing needs would put a nurse leader's skills strongly to the test. We'll say something about how you can learn to see with multiple perspectives later in the chapter.

• Do understand that you lead by how you are and who you are with every conversation you have. You need to be an authentic person because most people will spot very quickly where you are not. You need to walk your talk, not because your mother told you to, you learned it at school or your religion says you must. These may all be good reasons to walk your talk but the basic reason is that everyone will know if you don't! You may kid yourself that you can get away with the gap between what you say and what you do, but it will be a fantasy on your part. As a leader, it must be your sincere desire to know what it is like to be on the receiving end of your leadership. What is it like to be on the receiving end of me? It's a key question. You must gain a rounded sense of the answer.

• Do understand that your priority in all your work is to build relationships, to empower others, to create confidence, trust and positive energy. As well as sincere commitment to the work rooted in compassion, let there also be a spirit of play, of humour, a lightness of touch in your leadership. People own what they create. People want to know not only that they can have views, but that their views will count.

What do nurse and midwife leaders need to learn about culture?

Obviously we are not talking about culture as evoked by the image of the Royal Opera House in Covent Garden or the Summer Exhibition at the Royal Academy of Art. What you need as a nurse leader is the knowledge and skill to be able both to read and then influence your organisation's culture. In this sense of the word, a popular, informal definition of culture would be simply 'the way we do things around here'.

As we saw above, what we called 'the organisational environment' is not *fixed* in an organisation, so also the culture is not fixed. Ah, but it can get stuck.

Organisational cultures are powerful and the adage that 'Culture eats strategy for breakfast' can be all too true. If you had asked any of the nurses in the Mid Staffs hospital in the years when, as we now know, patient care sometimes amounted to a scandal, 'What quality of care would you want for your mother, your partner or your children?', what do you think they would have answered? We feel sure they would have wanted the best care for them (Ballatt and Campling, 2011). So how come good people like these, who want the best care, could get caught up in a culture where patients were drinking out of flower vases and sleeping in their own excrement? In short, it's because the culture had got stuck. So if we can see how this happened, and what you need to be aware of to prevent such a problem culture, we'll be a long way towards understanding what you need to do to make sure your culture is fit for purpose.

To set the context for thinking about organisational culture, it is once again useful to zoom out and see what's involved. We learn from sociology that all reality is socially constructed, the product of social, originally tribal, sense-making. As the French philosopher Pascal said, 'Truth on one side of the Pyrenees is error on the other'. Karl Marx, in his famous variation on this theme, showed how the vested interests of the powerful so forcibly affect the way a society lives its particular construction of reality. An example of what we take for granted but which is not 'objective reality' is noticeable in any BBC news bulletin. The focus of the news clearly draws the boundary around Britain and the British as being the obvious area of interest. That this is so seems obvious and natural and if the BBC gave as much attention to Africa as it does to Yorkshire we might well think it had lost the plot. The point is not whether the priorities of the BBC are suitable or not, it is that under examination they turn out to be *a choice*. It is not a given. It is not *objective* reality. The boundary of what interests us and what we care about could perfectly well be enlarged so that the top stories of the interdependent human family, rather than the national focus, became the norm.

Our evolutionary process
It is critical to note that modern human activity is the product of approximately 14 billion years of evolutionary process. We are hard-wired to survive. We have a reptilian brainstem that knows how to make us bite or fight or run away when we sense a threat to our survival. This has decisively affected the evolution of the human psyche. We may think our adult behaviour is all very civilised, polite and rational but as the eminient Austrian-British psychoanalyst Melanie Klein showed, our adult sophistications sit on a thin skin under which are seething, to use her language, all the depressive and persecutory anxieties we have carried since childhood (Klein, 1985). Klein explains that

these are not just properties of infancy – the urge to yell and scream when we're hurt, for example; they remain just under the surface all our lives. Protection and survival are, after all, paramount for a species. To survive, we have evolved a well-known series of ego defence mechanisms which protect us from the more unbearable and painful aspects of our existence. As T.S. Eliot (1974) wrote, 'Humankind cannot bear very much reality' (p. 178). Some of the ways in which we have evolved predispose us to seeing less than the full picture. We have individual blindspots. And we have social defences giving us collective or tribal blindspots. These start to matter when we don't notice that what we take for granted has aspects of bullying, scapegoating or persecution.

And of course, it follows from the point about the ubiquitous nature of human anxiety that we cannot afford to be rejected by our tribe. Our fear prevents us from stepping out of line. Our brain uses defences to rationalise what's going on around us. The research of Phil Zimbardo and many others shows how easily normally good people can become evil when their context changes (Zimbardo, 2007). Once outcast, our survival is at risk. So first we need to remember that human cultures are a product of human nature. We cannot buck our basic needs, as Abraham Maslow showed (1954). And one of those basic needs is for acceptance by our tribe. This predisposes us to accept the social norms all round us and this is a key factor in how cultures operate, as we shall see below.

Social norms and change blindness

The NHS is full of bright, intelligent people and, in 1990, a key priority was to stop working so much in silos and aim to work more collaboratively and corporately. But since then, not much has changed. It is as if different teams or departments unwittingly set up their own mini-tribes with their own norms and ways of doing things. Attitudes to taking breaks, punctuality, style of meetings, giving personal feedback, humour, commitment and a host of other variables can be so different even in adjacent departments. But silo working goes with a mentality that is really the opposite of systems thinking. Rather than exciting interest and curiosity in how other people are approaching things, silo working is closed to other perspectives. It prefers the familiar, the safe and the apparently 'known', however prejudiced and selective that 'knowledge'. And closely allied to silo working is conformist thinking. When we conform to the immediate social norms, we feel safer.

Take Zimbardo's well-known Stanford Prison experiment: After just a short time, student volunteer guards found themselves behaving brutally according to their imagined prison norms. Later, they said things like: 'I was surprised at myself … I made them call each other names and clean the toilet out with their bare hands. I practically considered the prisoners cattle …' or 'I was tired of seeing the prisoners in their rags and smelling them. I watched them tear at each other on orders given by us'. Or take the Milgram experiment at Yale University, repeated in many places all over the world with the same results. In the original experiment, it turned out that 65% of apparently perfectly normal people were willing to give what they thought were 450 volt fatal electric shocks to experimental subjects, in order to stay in line with expectations created in them by University staff (Milgram, 1974).

Put together, these experiments go a long way to explain not only how the situation that developed at Mid Staffs is all too possible, but how in any healthcare organisation, there is a constant risk of a drastic gap developing between espoused values and cultural norms. We like to think that we are individuals with a personal psychology that would never allow us to slip from the good of our upbringing, the values of our personal moral code and our beliefs. Unfortunately, repeated experiments reveal that only in rare and exceptional cases is the individual able to break from the social norms that their 'tribe' (silo, team, department, organisation, society) has developed around them. Think of Nazi Germany in the 1930s.

However, we are only 50% of the way to understanding a phenomenon like the Mid Staffs scandal. We need now to couple the almost unstoppable power of social norms with the equally potent force of what is called change blindness. This is the truth that when we are given something specific to focus on, we become blind to almost everything else. In Stafford it appears that prioritising certain targets like finance led to a remarkable blindness about the qulity of care. Though this reality is well evidenced, it is a shock to people when they find it applies to them! The best known example is the video clip in which a large gorilla walks through the middle of a group playing basketball. Those watching for the first time are asked to count the number of goals they see scored. Occupied by this task, a high percentage fail to notice the gorilla at all. When they are shown the clip a second time, they simply cannot believe they could have missed such a strong visual presence. Another famous example is the Door Study in which someone is asked to help give directions from a map. While they are talking together, two people carrying a large door pass between them and one of the door carriers exchanges places with the original person who asked for directions. They look different and are dressed differently but the man focused on giving directions is entirely oblivious of this swapover. They are many such studies all showing the same thing.

As a final example, seminary students in the USA were asked to prepare a school assembly on the parable of the Good Samaritan whose whole point was to encourage giving immediate help to someone in need. Each student was told to get a move on between the room they were in and the assembly hall because the children were waiting. In fact, the researchers had planted an apparently sick, groaning man in the corridor between the two spaces. Only 10% of the sudents stopped to help. When students were told there was no particular rush, then 63% stopped to help (Darley and Batson, 1973).

So when you add the power of social norms to the power of change blindness, and given the preoccupations of Stafford Hospital culture during the years of the scandal, you can see clearly how nurses who would want the best care for their nearest and dearest can become caught up in a culture that is promoting the opposite.

> How would you describe the culture of your team or your organisation? How could you influence this to create a culture that really works for you, your team, your organisation and of course your patients?

What do effective nurses need to understand, and to do, to promote best practice given these dangerous and ever-present forces?

- First, you need to be self-confident about your role. As a nurse, you are, please be reminded, a leader of the system.
- You need to claim the authority you legitimately have to be an architect of your culture.
- You have the right, indeed the duty, to analyse the culture of your organisation.
- You need to examine critically where it is fit for purpose and where it is going astray. So you need the skills of a cultural analyst. What environment should your culture be cultivating?
- You need to be one of those correcting and creating what the culture is becoming. You must make up your mind as to what the norms should be. Having decided, you need to influence the process of change.

What kind of culture is required to create the best care for patients and all staff?

When you have a good sense of this, you can analyse more critically.

- What do you need to keep from your culture and what needs to be changed? Then get a bit more subtle.
- The strategy and policies currently being adopted by your organisation – how far are they in alignment with your culture? Where are the gaps and what must be done to narrow them? What gets rewarded? This is important and must be observed and monitored closely.

- How consistently is alignment to best cultural values reinforced? How often is inappropriate cultural behaviour tolerated? This can be common, and of course the standard you walk past is the standard you accept. It can so easily become the case that an espoused high standard is more honoured in the breach than the observance.
- What about unintended consequences? Key performance indicators can be alerts as to what the organisation is focusing on. And that's where it is at risk of change blindness.

These are questions to think about in relation to the wider organisation. But each nurse leader has a responsibility to analyse their own behaviour and that of their immediate team. Everything you do and say, to use sociological parlance, is a signal. It points beyond itself. The signals you are generating matter enormously. They either promote the best organisational environment and culture or get in the way of the best.

One important practical task is to analyse your diary and daily calendar. Famously, calendars do not lie! If the story you tell yourself is that you are available but a diary analysis shows you spend a disproportionate amount of time in meetings, then your story is a self-deception. Your calendar needs to reflect the culture you believe in. An analysis can show how different what you spend your time on can be from what you would really prefer.

As a leader, one of your most useful resources is your imagination. Unfortunately, creative use of imagination is not relished anything like as much as it should and could be by most leaders. Do not let this be true in your case! How can you use your imagination to create a celebration, a welcome or farewell ceremony? How could you use visual images, symbols or cartoons to increase the impact of communication? How can you illustrate important messages to make them more memorable? What else can you imagine doing to enable more participation in any aspect of the work? How can you promote everyone's sense of a common vision and identity. Remember the three key questions when considering a rebrand. What do we stand for? What makes us stand out? What makes us compelling?

Finally, be imaginative about rules and keep them simple. Take a leaf out of the giant American company Nordstrom. They only have one rule for all staff. It is this: 'use your best judgement'.

In conclusion, your aim and duty as a leader is to analyse your culture and then be an agent of cultural change to shape your culture positively for the patient. Look at the Culture Web (see Figure 4.1 in Chapter 4) to help your analysis. You will know when you have developed the mindset of a leader and are thinking with a systems perspective when you have:

- given up the fantasy that you can control other human beings
- given up trying to control the variables in a wicked problem

- started, instead, to build relationships around the core purpose and values of the organisation
- started to empower others to get involved in a co-created vision of best practice
- started to trust that when work is rooted in humane values, expressed in a co-created vision which everyone owns and is repeatedly talked about, you have the makings of a sustainable system and a positive culture.

References

Ballatt, J. and Campling, P. (2011) *Intelligent Kindness: reforming the culture of healthcare.* London: Royal College of Psychiatrists.

Chapman, J. (2002) *System Failure: why governments must learn to think differently.* London: Demos.

Darley, J.M. and Batson, C.D. (1973) From Jerusalem to Jericho. A study of situational and dispositional variables in helping behaviour. *Journal of Personality & Social Psychology,* 27(1), 100–108.

Eliot, T.S. (1974) *Collected Poems 1909–1962.* London: Faber and Faber.

Goleman, D. (1996) *Emotional Intelligence: why it can matter more than IQ.* London: Bloomsbury.

Gribbin, J. (1984) *In Search of Schrodinger's Cat: quantum physics and reality.* New York: Bantam.

Grint, K. (2010) *Leadership: a very short introduction.* Oxford: Oxford University Press.

Heifetz, R. and Linsky, M. (2002) *Leadership on the Line: staying alive through the dangers of leading.* Boston, MA: Harvard Business School Press.

Klein, M. (1985) Our adult world and its roots in infancy. In: Coleman, A.D. and Geller, M.H. (eds) *Group Relations Reader 2.* Washington, DC: A.K. Rice Institute, pp. 5–19.

Maslow, A. (1954) *Motivation and Personality.* New York: Harper.

Milgram, S. (1974) *Obedience to Authority: an experimental view.* London: Tavistock Publications.

Stokes, K.M. (1995) *Paradigm Lost: a cultural and systems theoretical critique of political economy.* New York: M.E. Sharpe.

Wheatley, M.J. (1999) *Leadership and the New Science: discovering order in a chaotic world.* San Francisco, CA: Berrett-Koehler.

Zimbardo, P.G. (2007) *The Lucifer Effect: understanding how good people turn evil.* New York: Random House.

Chapter 9 Helping to lead the NHS into the future

Caroline Alexander, Catherine Eden, Nichole McIntosh, Natilla Henry with David Ashton, Michelle Mello

In the final chapter of this book, we have asked a range of people to give their perspective on what the future holds for nursing and midwifery. Contributors have commented on compassion and the need to be truly inclusive in terms of how we deliver care as well as how well we engage with each other. They also speak about the 'value-quality-finance' equation and the importance of nurses and midwives engaging with and being a visibly positive force in relation to 'large P' politics as well as the 'small p' politics of daily organisational life, something which the majority of this book addresses.

The contributors have articulated their ideas about the future in different ways. So in addition to providing a crucially important view from a political and strategic perspective, others have recounted their very personal journeys and their opinions of what the future might hold. One of the authors speaks about the future of nursing being in the hands of the many; we all have a responsibility for it and are custodians of it. Another account is in the form of a semi-structured conversation with one of the book's editors on the impact of positive role models, whilst the final piece in the chapter is in the form of a letter from the writer as she is now to her younger self – a letter of wisdom, guidance and love.

Strategy, systems and compassion

Caroline Alexander

When I was asked to contribute to this book, I thought it would be easy to describe what we need in nurse leaders of the future. I had many ideas in my head built up from my own experiences, frustrations and reading, reflections on learning from colleagues both within nursing and more widely, and

How to be a Nurse or Midwife Leader, First Edition.
Edited by David Ashton, Jamie Ripman and Philippa Williams.
© 2017 John Wiley & Sons, Ltd. Published 2017 by John Wiley & Sons, Ltd.

those I mentor. However, the complex world we live in, with the many new opportunities of the Five Year Forward View and the operational challenges experienced by all delivering healthcare today, made this a much more challenging task than I anticipated! I could have written a thesis but have decided to focus on three key leadership behaviours/priorities which I believe we haven't capitalised on enough as a profession and which we need to address as leaders if we are to really add value.

Strategic clinical leadership across systems and geographies that span organisational boundaries

To meet the value, quality and finance challenge, to be really effective nurse leaders need to be visible, active clinical leaders, not just nursing leaders and not just leaders within their own sphere of influence or organisation. If nurse leaders are not at the table when new clinical strategies are being developed, great opportunities will be missed in terms of creativity in models of care and staffing. This needs to happen at all levels of nursing, whether it is designing new ways of delivering care on wards, maximising the contribution of the whole multidisciplinary team to secure value, developing new care pathways across organisational boundaries locally, supporting parity of esteem between mental and physical health or a COPD pathway, getting the best out of specialist and generalist roles, or reconfiguring health services across large geographies. If we aren't around the table from the beginning, we will always be the add-on. It is not always easy to be heard but the more nurse leaders can network across geographies that make sense to them, the bigger impact we can have.

Strategic professional leadership

To me, this is about developing a sound evidence base for professional practice and then collective debate and agreement as a profession when practice needs to change. We as nurse leaders need to engage in the debate and take ownership, otherwise the decisions will be made by others, which won't be good for patients, the profession or us as individuals. By this, I don't mean stick always to what we know but open our eyes and ears to new ideas and also understand that we must consider the unintended consequence of change and if something isn't safe, have the courage to fight for it. We are at a time, more than ever before, when we need to work collaboratively to respond to the pressures we face, whether that is working collaboratively to secure recruitment, for example the Capital Nurse programme across London, or development of bridging roles and making sure what is decided on is workable in both the short and long term. On another note, we know how easy it is to stay in our comfort zone. We need to be willing to step between commissioning, provision, system leadership and academia throughout our careers to keep the debate fresh and ensure that nursing across all parts of the system is equally valued. I have done that throughout my career and am about to make another transition. I believe it has added to my breadth of insight, confidence and ability to influence as a leader.

Collective, compassionate leaders

We all talk about delivering compassionate care to our patients and that nurses are the guardians of this. To deliver truly compassionate care to our patients, what does that mean for how we treat our own staff? Through action area 4 of the Compassion in Practice strategy, I have had the opportunity to look at the role leadership and culture play in how we deliver compassionate care. All I can say is, we underestimate it at our peril. We commissioned some research – *Building and Strengthening Leadership: Leading with Compassion* (www.england.nhs.uk/wp-content/uploads/2014/12/london-nursing-accessible.pdf) – with a supporting field guide which looked at leadership for compassion through a range of lenses and reflects the views of frontline leaders. The field guide is particularly useful for those days when you are struggling or reflecting as it gives you insight into what derails you and what enables your leadership.

Listening to our staff and valuing their contribution have never been more important. The work of Michael West and colleagues really demonstrates that this is critical. New models like Buurtzorg which are being considered for implementation in the UK require a different type of leadership – empowering the front line to make decisions and self-governing teams with evidence-based outcomes. This is uncomfortable for a system that is designed as a hierarchy – how do we learn to let go and trust?

Finally, how we treat BME nurses and midwives and the opportunity we give them are things that the profession needs to take seriously. We *all* must step up and be role models in how we support staff from BME backgrounds to take their rightful place in the leadership of the NHS.

Conclusion

In summary, you could say these three areas apply to all disciplines and not just nursing. Yes they do but we need to be role models and grasp this time of opportunity if we are to make sure that nursing is centre stage and making a real difference to the health of the population of England and beyond.

We are fortunate to have some of the most creative and innovative leaders within our profession. We need to harness them and enable them to have as big an impact as possible and minimise the blocks that get in the way. We don't have a very structured career framework once people qualify, unlike other disciplines; this is a blessing in many ways but also a curse. A blessing in that it enables a breadth of insight and approach built up of different experiences; I can attest to that from my own career. But a curse because we cannot guarantee consistency when it comes to learning to be an executive director, for instance, and the pressure that can place on individuals when they first step up to those types of roles.

I am going to leave you with some questions.

- If we are to be strategic clinical and nursing leaders who are inclusive and compassionate, what does that mean for the preparation of nurses both undergraduate and postgraduate?
- How do we help ourselves?

Work with others to influence the politics, with a small and a large P

Catherine Eden

For many people, when the word 'politics' is mentioned, their eyes glaze over and they think of politicians in Westminster shouting at each other at Prime Minister's Question Time. However, nurses and midwives, from students to the Chief Nurse, have long been involved in influencing and shaping the health system for patients, as well as the role and working practices of nurses.

We hope this book will inspire, motivate and give you the confidence to get involved to make a difference to the things that matter to you and your patients, whether you are a student or a newly qualified nurse or are taking on a new leadership role. Being more politically astute is not something to be feared and the ostrich approach to politics in all its forms – sticking your head in the sand – is never going to be a successful one.

Often nurses may feel that they don't have the power to change things, but with around 692 000 nurses on the NMC register, this couldn't be less true. At the 2015 general election, the RCN highlighted the fact that there are around 1800 nurses living in each parliamentary constituency and the difference their votes could make to the result.

When thinking about politics in its widest form and influencing for change, it is worth starting with the question, 'Where does the power lie and who has the power to make the change you are wanting?'. It can be helpful to start the process by putting together a 'power map', with the problem or thing you would like to change at the centre, then brainstorming the many people that could have an influence on solving that problem or who might have a part to play in giving the result that you want. For example, if you wanted to change the shift patterns of your team because you felt that the changeover times were not good for patients, you would start by thinking about all the people who may have an influence over successfully making the changes you believe to be right. You then have a group of people with whom you need to work and influence to effect change.

When thinking about power, it is worth bearing in mind that power often lies in surprising places; it might be the GP receptionist who holds the key to making referrals for patients run more smoothly, or a patient and carer group that has the most influence over improving outpatient flows. It is thus worth looking at where your existing links are with those individuals who are the key to change and who is more likely to be able to successfully influence them.

So, you've decided what you want to change or highlight and have mapped the array of people who can help you achieve that. What next? It is then time to think about:

- WHO do you want to target?
- What MESSAGES do you want to convey?
- What ACTION are you asking for?
- WHO is best placed to make the approach?

For most nurses and midwives, becoming more engaged with the politics of health in all its forms is about building a system that works in the interests of patients and for the nursing staff who serve them. But this can be a daunting prospect for many nurses as common thoughts about politics include 'it's too complicated', 'they won't listen anyway', 'I can't do anything to make a difference'.

For many years, campaigning for change has revolved around writing letters, attending marches and gathering awareness and support through print and broadcast media. But the world has changed dramatically since the arrival of social media and there are now many more ways in which nurses can campaign, influence and highlight areas for change. Examples on Twitter such as @WeNurses and @WeMidwives and @britainsnurses give a forum for nurses and midwives to find like-minded colleagues all over the world and discuss issues of concern. Social media campaigns such as #stopthepressure and the highly successful #hellomynameis can spread health and care messages widely and gather support for change. The creative use of Facebook and other platforms for spreading messages and gathering support is increasingly important. Organisations such as 38 Degrees can be a good way to gain support for a particular change and there are various petition websites that can be an effective way to highlight local, national and international issues. The use of social media is also a great way to talk to people that in the normal course of your day you wouldn't come across, be they politicians, media outlets or those who run the organisations you work for. Some of the country's nursing leaders, such as Jane Cummings, Viv Bennett, Janet Davies and Lisa Bayliss-Pratt, are great users of social media and getting involved allows you to 'speak' to them in a way that might not be possible otherwise.

Big P politics

Before running a fringe meeting at a recent nursing conference, we asked around 15 current and former MPs and peers the first three words that came into their mind about nurses. Answers ranged from 'admired and greatly valued profession' and 'underpaid and put upon' to 'not what they were' and 'limited confidence'. Around 50% of the comments were positive and the other half were less so.

It is interesting to note that in Parliament, there are only a handful of former nurses across both the House of Commons and the House of Lords and so the opinions that national politicians have of nurses and nursing today are often formed from assumptions, rather than from fact.

If you are looking to make changes that require the support of local or national MPs, the first challenge is to help those politicians understand what modern nursing is ... and what it isn't. The same would apply if you were looking to influence elected local councillors, Members of the Scottish Parliament, Welsh and London Assemblies, and the Northern Ireland Executive.

The second thing is to consider the people you are trying to influence and here are some top tips that we hope will help. But the most important thing is to start the conversation.

Top 10 tips for working successfully with politicians

1 Where does the power lie and who has the power to change things? Pick who you want to influence carefully.

2 Know your politician: how interested are they in health; how do they like to receive information; what are they saying in local/social media; what committees/groups are they on; what is their majority and where are they in the electoral cycle?

3 Establish relations in good times and ensure regular contact if appropriate. Remember that for all politicians, be they local, regional or national, the constituents who vote for them are their number 1 priority.

4 Most politicians are generalists, dealing with many issues; health is just one, albeit important, part of their job. 'Local' is also important; interest will be higher if the issue is about local people or services, or about national/international factors that will have a local impact.

5 Evidence-based information is appreciated; aim for it to be concise, appropriate and relevant. Find out how they prefer to receive information – written, email, in person.

> **6** Handle politicians with care and maintain your political independence, especially around election time; don't get caught between 'the dog and the lamp post'.
>
> **7** Have a small number of clear messages and be specific on what action you would like the politician to take.
>
> **8** Don't assume they talk to other local politicians, even when in the same party, or that councillors talk to their local MPs and vice versa. There may be great links between politicians in the same area, or there may not. Sometimes politicians from different parties will work together if it is first and foremost a local matter.
>
> **9** Politicians are people people. Tell stories, show projects and invite them to your workplaces or to meet affected patients and staff. It's really powerful.
>
> **10** The photo opportunity. Think about joint opportunities for media activity – traditional and social media.

Resources

www.nmc.org.uk/contact-us/

www.hsj.co.uk/topics/technology-and-innovation/it-started-with-a-tweet-how-social-media-sparked-a-campaign-for-change/5078128.article

Compassion and cultural competence

Nichole McIntosh

Nursing on the frontline, or coalface, as it can often feel like, has never been an easy occupational choice. Indeed, I can remember being repeatedly told by my lecturers during my pre-registration nursing training programme 15 years ago that nursing is a vocation and that you do it because you are passionate about caring for patients and not for the money. To be frank, nursing is not for everyone. It takes a special person with compassion, kindness and selflessness to be a good nurse.

The counterbalance of this view of nursing being a challenging career choice is the high esteem in which the nursing profession was held in society. The caricature of nurses as angels was prominent in the media. You simply had to mention that you were a nurse and immediately barriers were broken down and trust and confidence in what you said and did were assured.

Unfortunately, over the years, there has been an unmistakable erosion of public trust and confidence in nurses and the image of nursing as a trustworthy and caring profession has taken a significant hit. Anecdotal and media reports of nurses behaving inappropriately towards vulnerable patients and at times willfully harming patients have resulted in public trust and confidence in nurses being at an all-time low. There have been national campaigns to raise awareness of the invaluable role that nurses continue to play in keeping patients healthy and safe at some of the most stressful times of their lives. The emphasis of these campaigns has overwhelmingly been on assuring the public that providing 'basic' or 'fundamental' care with compassion and promoting the dignity of all patients remain the priorities of the nursing profession. The image of nursing is still being resuscitated and there is some way to go before it could be viewed as being universally respected as it once was.

The future of nursing as a profession is in my view positive. We are at a crossroads and must act now to ensure the future remains positive. There are green shoots of change in recognising the value of diversity in the nursing workforce to enable the provision of culturally competent and compassionate care. The case for having a workforce that reflects the communities that they serve has been well made and is being gradually accepted. There has been a paradigm shift which has led to an increased range of programmes available to ensure that there are equal opportunities for professional and career development of all nursing staff, including those from black and minority ethnic backgrounds.

However, there are still challenges which must be overcome to safeguard the future of the nursing profession and improve the standards that we hold so dear. Safeguarding the future of nursing as a profession will undoubtedly require courageous nursing leaders who are prepared to stand unequivocally against a culture of poor standards of care and failure, bullying, unsafe staffing levels and discrimination against staff based on any of the protected equality and diversity characteristics of the Equality and Human Rights Commission.

Role modelling of the compassionate, caring nurse must be evident from the Board to the ward. Senior nursing leaders need to be visible, accessible, approachable and, most importantly, trustworthy. Frontline staff need to be assured that the senior leaders will 'walk the talk' and are passionate about providing an environment in which patients, relatives and staff have positive experiences of care. The culture of an organisation is set at the top. The care standards and expectations of behaviour start at Board level and are filtered through every layer of management and to the frontline staff. 'The standard you walk past is the standard you accept.' Never has this been truer than in promoting the future of nursing. We have to create a culture of nursing practice in which we would be proud to be a patient. Forget the friends and family test, would *we* choose to be treated at our place of work?

The future of nursing is in the hands of the nurse leaving nursing college. It is in the hands of the nurse who has five, 10, 15 or even 30 years experience.

In fact, the future of nursing is in the hands of anyone who has been privileged enough to earn the title of registered nurse. It *is* a privilege and an honour to be assessed as being of good character and to be worthy of being called 'nurse'. We must treasure that privilege and do whatever is required to ensure that no-one, absolutely no-one is allowed to destroy it.

An emotional connection 200 miles apart

Natilla Henry and David Ashton
We set out to write a piece for this section of the book based on the outputs of a semi-structured interview, with David interviewing Natilla about her experiences in leadership, what had motivated her and what words of advice she might give to someone moving into a leadership role. In part, we stayed with that approach, but out of that process a quite spontaneous and unexpected emotional connection happened even though we were on the other end of a phone line and 200 miles apart.

Firstly, though, here is an abridged version of our semi-structured conversation.

> **David:** *What do you think brought you to be in a leadership role in midwifery?*
>
> **Natilla:** *I think there were two things really. Firstly, it felt like a natural step born out of expectation. At the time you tended to move through your career in what might be seen as a predictable way – from student, to qualification, through various grades to a position of clinical leadership. The options would then tend to be a move into lecturing or management. Secondly was a personal ambition – I wanted to be a leader one day to make positive changes to midwifery, not sitting back and being done to but by making a positive contribution.*
>
> **David:** *What words of guidance would you give to someone early in their career as a midwife?*
>
> **Natilla:** *I think I would take that back even further – there is something about the expectations of someone entering midwifery as a career. It is a career, role, vocation to be proud of, and it's hard. If your expectation is not realistic coming into the role, you could be disappointed or disaffected; this doesn't help anyone. You will need resilience and to develop that you need support around you. Although midwifery training is a university degree, it is fundamentally about being with a woman. You need to be altruistic, you need to be able to set yourself aside in the service of the other – you need to be prepared to, and able to, give of yourself. Network*

and develop the support of like-minded people to make sure you have that support to develop your resilience ... AND enjoy the journey. As well as some hard situations, you will see and experience much that is positive from the women and families you will work alongside – the life you have played a part in bringing into the world – this will compensate for some of the hard times.

David: *What words of advice would you give for those people moving into more formal leadership roles within the profession?*

Natilla: *The type of people who generally come into midwifery are looking to work with the woman and her family. They then move up the ranks into managerial and leadership roles – they can end up in a leadership role without any formal training or development. You need to get some* [development]. *You are entering a political climate – yes you need to be a clinical expert, but that isn't enough on its own. Because of the need to be very focused on the woman, unborn or newly born child and the family, and rightly so, you need to start looking much more widely. You need to avoid being insular – for example, not all women are healthy so you will need to work with other professions and AHPs* [allied health professionals] *for support with other physical and psychological conditions.*

The clinical grounding you have is important, your core values and remembering what midwifery is all about matter – remember that. You will also need to be flexible without losing your integrity – remember your core purpose. There is a need to be creative, develop innovative solutions, offer alternatives to complex situations – if you don't, others may impose something.

Above all, working in midwifery offers a great opportunity, yes you need to be resilient, embrace it!

So now back to the emotional connection. During our conversation, Natilla recalled people who had been significant to her in her career. There was no one person who came to mind immediately until she remembered a midwifery tutor she'd had, a woman called Janet Blake who, like Natilla, has Caribbean ancestry. Natilla recounted the occasion when she first encountered Janet and that at the end of the session, she couldn't recall a word that Janet had said, yet had been totally caught up in the experience of her presence. Janet's passion, a word sometimes used glibly, had been so present that it connected with an aspect of Natilla. In effect, the essence of Janet's passion had connected very deeply with an aspect of Natilla's self which until that point had been dormant. That emotional connection had carried over the years as part of Natilla's sense of herself as a midwife, and although David was 200 miles away from Natilla, at the other end of the phone line having never met Janet, in that moment that essence was transmitted. Our reflection on this experience was that we sometimes need to revisit who we are today as a result of what happened yesterday, as this makes us the people we might be for tomorrow.

Enjoy every moment, never stop learning and don't ever forget why you came into nursing

Michelle Mello

From:
   Michelle Mello
   Deputy Director of Nursing
   NHS England

To:
   Michelle Mello
   First Year Student Nurse
   University of Hull

June 2016

Hi Michelle,

Re: From Michelle at 49 to Michelle at 18 – the Voice of Experience!

Yes it's you! 31 years later. Still in nursing, you made it! Hooray! Still enjoying it. Here are some top tips on how to be a great nurse. Who knows where that may lead you...

Listen to others carefully, Michelle, it's not as easy as it sounds, but you will learn so much. I know you think you can change the world right now (never stop believing this!) but always take time to listen, observe and learn from others. You will learn lots about kindness and compassion from amazing nurses, nursing assistants, clinicians and support staff you will work with and encounter. From patients and their families; they understand themselves and often their illness better than you, so always see the patient as an equal, if not an expert. Listen to them and treat them as you want to be treated yourself.

You will also meet and learn from some great nurse leaders; remember that they are human so don't be frightened to engage. Display the behaviours you admire in them and strive to be a great role model yourself. Of course, you will also observe some behaviour that you will not want to copy; don't forget this too! Every nurse is a leader and has the potential to impact on the people in their care and those around them. Leadership isn't about seniority, it's about behaviour, so never underestimate the impact of your behaviour on others. As the great Maya Angelou said, 'People will forget what you said, people will forget what you did, but people will never forget how you made them feel'.

You are going to love being a nurse, Michelle, and you've chosen the right career. You will meet, work with and care for some amazing people along the way. You will learn lots about various clinical and health-related subjects and also learn a lot about yourself. You will learn what it takes to be a good nurse leader. It's a real privilege to be a nurse. Never forget that and as you progress, always remember what it was like at the start.

Theory and research are really, really important. I know that you can't wait to get your hands on people and be a 'real nurse' but understanding the reasons behind what you do and how you make decisions should always have a sound evidence base. It will influence how you practise for the rest of your career. One day you may even get to meet some of the early nurse researchers you studied! There are going to be some amazing changes in how we connect and engage with others which will happen over the next few decades – but that's another story …

As a 'university nurse', people will judge you as being different. You already have experience of being different, being a black, working-class girl from Liverpool! Being different can bring its own challenges and make it hard to fit in, but it also gives you the opportunity to help others see that being different can be a positive thing and that underneath it we are all human and have things in common. It's a reminder that we should all celebrate diversity. Never forget your roots and don't be afraid to be you. Some of the best nurses and leaders you will meet are genuine, humble and not afraid to be vulnerable at times.

The journey will not always be easy. You are going to come across people, situations and obstacles (assignments and exams are just the start!) that will test your reserves, self-belief and emotions. Nurses are there for people at the best and worst of times, so expect some big emotional moments along the way. Dig deep, turn to your family and friends and never forget your values. Hold them dear, be strong and resilient. You will be fine in the end, honestly! Everyone makes mistakes; what distinguishes a great nurse is how you learn from them.

This brings me to an important point. Look after yourself physically, emotionally and mentally. I know you are young, fit and full of life but do set aside time for yourself. Treasure your family, friends and colleagues and don't be afraid to ask for help when you need it. Relationships and networks are so vital and you will learn who to trust and who to let go. Trust your instincts but don't be surprised if you get it wrong sometimes.

Don't be afraid to take chances with your career - nothing ventured, nothing gained. Dream big, chase your dreams and don't let anyone tell you that things aren't possible. You are going to achieve great things! A top tip is to remember that although lots of care goes on in hospitals, there is a whole world of health and care outside of them in primary care, the community, research and teaching so don't limit your options or thinking about where you may work next.

One of the most rewarding things you can do is to help others beyond people/patients you will care for. There will be chances to teach, develop and share your learning with others so grab them.

Getting through university and qualifying is the start of your amazing journey. Study hard but have fun too! Of course, the grade you achieve matters to you right now but hardly anyone will ask you about it in the future.

Make the most of it, Michelle, I know you will. Enjoy every moment, never stop learning and don't ever forget why you came into nursing in the first place.

Good luck,
Michelle xx

Afterword

David Ashton, Jamie Ripman and Philippa Williams

We started writing this book in April 2015. Over a year later, we are about to submit the final draft to the publisher, and by the time you read this it will probably be a further year down the line.

As we say in the introduction, the beginnings of the book came from the programmes run by the NHS Leadership Academy. Since we started, many of the participants on those programmes will have changed roles, moved organisations, developed further as leaders, and continued to make wonderful and significant contributions to patient care and the development of the NHS for the future. In May 2016, Professor Jane Cummings, Chief Nursing Officer for England, launched the new strategy for nursing, midwifery and care staff, *Leading Change, Adding Value*, which explicitly focuses on the key leadership contribution of nursing, midwifery and care staff to influence and lead improvement in patient care and outcomes. And since we started writing, there have been many other significant events in the healthcare sector and in wider society and by the time you read this, there will probably have been even more. Change is a constant and part of any leadership role is to be able to respond to the evolving context in which we find ourselves.

We would like to end with some examples of the changes some of the participants have made as a result of deliberately and intentionally choosing to develop their leadership, to experiment with different approaches, to build their self-awareness and confidence. They are a few out of many such that demonstrate how nurse leaders have brought their passion, skill and commitment to bear to make a difference to staff and patients.

How to be a Nurse or Midwife Leader, First Edition.
Edited by David Ashton, Jamie Ripman and Philippa Williams.
© 2017 John Wiley & Sons, Ltd. Published 2017 by John Wiley & Sons, Ltd.

You see, the future is in your hands! We hope this book will help support you on the way.

'*At the end of the course I was promoted to Matron. I am now more involved in meetings and my opinions are being voiced. I also help others in our team with group discussions and actively listen to their concerns and take any necessary action required.*'

'*I have joined the staff engagement group and hope to make a difference with this group. I am getting together a support group for matrons based on the impact groups from the leadership course.*'

'*I have made loads of changes. I ran a rapid change fortnight last summer out of which we developed an acuity process to aid patient flow through the emergency pathway [bed allocation tool]; adapted our falls prevention plan and achieved a 40% reduction in high harm falls; plus lots of other changes that have impacted on patient care.*'

'*I have changed the culture of the service I lead, developed mentorship opportunities, set a clear direction and can see how differently staff treat each other and therefore our families.*'

'*I am working in the CCG to transform the way nursing services are delivered in the community; I have been selling the idea of a nurse who can work across district and GP surgeries to deliver LTC care to house-bound people. This has meant negotiating the role with the CCG then per-suading them to invest, then setting up the pilot. I am in negotiation with a local university to commission an accredited level 6–7 course for this. I have also persuaded local nurses to pilot NMC revalidation, set up local action learning sets to add to CPD and am hoping to start a doctor-ate looking at the professionalisation of nursing.*'

'*I have been able to take a step back from my job and reflect on what I really want to achieve and what my core values are in what I do. I now find myself saying "but what does this mean for patients?" more often.*'

'*I became a much better leader and my team appreciated this; this also reflected in the care patients received from staff. I am now working on a large change programme and using the skills I developed on the programme to do this.*'

'*Team benefits – improved morale, sickness and absence, productivity. Patients – improved discharge processes – leading to reduced length of stay.*'

'*I am a stronger leader and have greater faith in my abilities. As a result, I have stood up for what I believe in and implemented change across my professional remit. I am encouraging my Matrons to do the same and prioritise patient care above all else.*'

'*Personally – huge benefit came at a time when I was feeling undervalued and not sure of future career options. Regained my confidence and have successfully been appointed to a new more senior role which has accountability for nursing leadership and quality of care.*'

'*Complaints have gone down and my service has a reputation for excellent delivery of care. We are aware of our risk areas and are proactive about them. We are learning how to challenge each other constructively to get the best from each other. This has changed from a culture of suspicion and negativity. Staff who did not deliver the best care have left as there was a clear message of addressing poor performance.*'

'*I found that becoming a leader is more about understanding ourselves. I had read some of Daniel Goleman's stuff on Emotional Intelligence and really wanted to be that sort of leader. So I began to practise NOT jumping in with a solution but becoming aware of how knowing myself helped me to know how others felt about or viewed situations. I have always found negative people difficult to deal with; people who cannot immediately grasp the advantages really annoy me. During and since the course I have been able, not only to see points of view, but patiently accept starting where other people actually are. I have led the recent NMC revalidation pilot in our CCG and had to spend a lot of time "holding hands" with anxious nurses. This time has paid dividends as 88% of piloteers completed the challenge, many to a very high standard, and are now, by their own admission, confident and prepared for the real thing.*'

Index

How to be a Nurse or Midwife Leader, First Edition.
Edited by David Ashton, Jamie Ripman and Philippa Williams.
© 2017 John Wiley & Sons, Ltd. Published 2017 by John Wiley & Sons, Ltd.